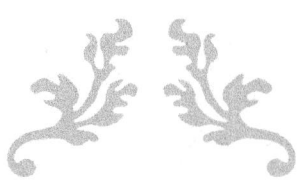

AI REVOLUTION IN MEDICINE & HEALTHCARE

Digital Transformation through Artificial Intelligence

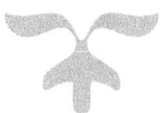

DECEMBER 23, 2024
JAYANT DESHMUKH

Disclaimer

The information provided in this book is for general informational and educational purposes only. Every effort has been made to ensure the accuracy and reliability of the content at the time of publication. However, the author and publisher make no representations or warranties regarding the completeness, accuracy, or suitability of the information contained in this book.

The tools, applications, and techniques mentioned are subject to changes in availability, pricing, and functionality by their respective developers or organizations. Readers are advised to conduct their own research and exercise discretion before using any tool or implementing any recommendations.

The author and publisher shall not be held liable for any damages, losses, or adverse consequences arising from the use or misuse of the information provided herein. Any reliance you place on the information in this book is strictly at your own risk.

This book includes references to third-party tools, websites, and applications, which are used solely for informational purposes. The inclusion of such references does not imply endorsement or

Copyright @2024 Jayant Deshmukh

affiliation with the respective developers or organizations.

This book does not serve as financial, legal, or technical advice. For specific concerns or personalized recommendations, readers are encouraged to consult professionals in the relevant fields.

By reading this book, you acknowledge that you have read, understood, and agree to the terms of this disclaimer.

AI REVOLUTION IN MEDICINE AND HEALTHCARE: DIGITAL TRANSFORMATION THROUGH ARTIFICIAL INTELLIGENCE

First edition. December 23, 2024.
Copyright © 2024 Jayant Deshmukh.
Written by Jayant Deshmukh.

Copyright @2024 Jayant Deshmukh

Table of Contents

About the Author 5
Prologue 9
Introduction 14
Chapter 1: The Current State of Healthcare and Medicine 21
Chapter 2: Demystifying Artificial Intelligence in Healthcare .. 28
Chapter 3: AI in Diagnostics and Imaging 36
Chapter 4: AI in Drug Discovery and Development 43
Chapter 5: AI in Personalized Medicine 51
Chapter 6: AI in Surgery and Robotics 59
Chapter 7: AI in Preventive Healthcare and Wellness 66
Chapter 8: AI in Patient Engagement and Experience 73
Chapter 9: AI in Healthcare Administration and Operations .. 81
Chapter 10: AI in Global Health and Public Health Challenges 89
Chapter 11: Ethical and Regulatory Challenges in AI-Driven Healthcare 96
Chapter 12: Future of AI in Medicine and Healthcare 103
Chapter 13: The Human Side of AI in Healthcare 111
Chapter 14: Inspiring Stories and Success Cases 122
Chapter 15: How AI is Benefiting Humanity 129
Conclusion 138
Glossary of Terms 144
References 145

Copyright @2024 Jayant Deshmukh

A Personal Message to You 148

Copyright @2024 Jayant Deshmukh

About the Author

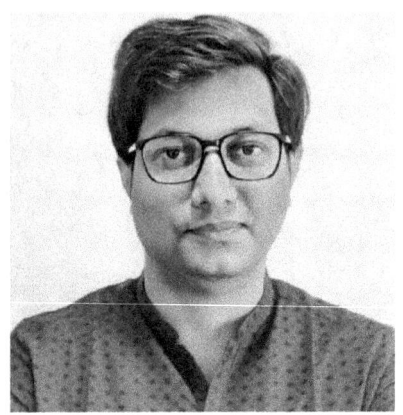

Jayant Deshmukh is a visionary leader at the intersection of technology and human potential. A Certified Project Management Professional (PMP) and an accomplished AI practitioner, Jayant has an extensive career spanning over one and half decades. His expertise lies in orchestrating complex **digital transformation initiatives** for banks and financial institutions across the globe.

Jayant's journey is marked by a unique blend of professional excellence and cultural immersion. Having traveled to and worked in multiple countries, he possesses a deep understanding of diverse geographies, cultures, and societal dynamics. This exposure has enabled him to navigate global challenges effectively while empathizing with people's unique personas and needs. His ability to blend technical know-how with a nuanced appreciation of human behavior has been a cornerstone of his success in both corporate and social spheres.

Beyond his professional endeavors, Jayant is passionately committed to **social causes**. He has actively engaged with communities to understand the challenges of the common man and develop tech-driven initiatives to address issues like unemployment, education, and access to healthcare. His ability to see the human side of technology makes his work relatable and impactful.

Books Authored by Jayant Deshmukh

Jayant has penned several impactful books that reflect his expertise, passion, and vision for empowering individuals and professionals. Each book is crafted with a human touch, engaging storytelling, and actionable insights.

1. **Prompt Engineering - The Ultimate Guide for Success in Artificial Intelligence**

This definitive guide to AI prompt engineering offers a comprehensive introduction to AI interaction, helping both beginners and professionals harness AI's power. Packed with practical tools, insights, and examples, it empowers readers to leverage AI effectively in their daily and professional lives.

2. **Mastering the Art of Corporate Communication**

Aimed at enhancing influence, collaboration, and leadership, this book explores 149 effective communication strategies essential for success in the corporate world. It provides actionable advice and real life examples, equipping readers to strengthen their communication skills and make an impact in any professional setting.

3. **Step by Step Guide to Overcome Corporate Politics**

Through a practical and storytelling-driven approach, this book presents 105 proven techniques to navigate and resolve corporate politics. It helps readers manage office dynamics, avoid conflicts, and thrive in their professional journeys, all while maintaining authenticity and integrity.

4. **Digital Transformation in Banking & Finance:** Unlocking the Power of 110 AI Tools to Revolutionize the Banking and Finance Industry An in-depth exploration of how AI tools are transforming the banking and finance sectors, this book provides insights into 110 AI-powered tools that enhance productivity, improve customer experiences, and drive innovation. It's a must-read for financial professionals looking to embrace AI.

5. **Building a Career in AI: A Practical Guide for Aspiring Professionals** A motivational and inspiring guide for individuals starting or transitioning into AI careers. This book offers real-life examples, practical advice, and actionable steps, serving as a roadmap for aspiring AI professionals to succeed in this dynamic field.

6. **AI Tools for Everyone: 119 Best AI Tools to Master Everyday Tasks** This book introduces readers to 119 AI tools designed to improve efficiency and productivity in everyday tasks. From personal use to business applications, Jayant demonstrates how these tools simplify processes and help users accomplish more in less time, making AI accessible to all.

7. **10x Productivity Hacks: Unlocking the Secrets of AI to Boost Productivity, Efficiency and Transform Your Life** A practical guide that shares powerful strategies and tools to dramatically enhance productivity. It offers actionable insights for individuals looking to maximize their output while maintaining a healthy work-life balance.

8. **Nurturing Growth Mindset: A Parent's Guide for Raising Innovative, Adaptive and Empowered Children** This book is a heartfelt guide for parents, blending Jayant's professional acumen with his personal experiences as a parent. It

offers insights into equipping children with the skills, resilience, and mindset needed to thrive in the AI-driven world.

Through his books, Jayant Deshmukh continues to inspire, educate, and empower readers to embrace technology and innovation as tools for personal and professional growth. His writing is a reflection of his belief that **technology is not just about advancement—it's about enhancing the human experience.**

Connect with Jayant Deshmukh on social media at :

https://www.instagram.com/jayantdeshmukhofficial/

https://www.linkedin.com/in/jayant-deshmukh-pmp/

https://www.facebook.com/jayantdeshmukh01

https://www.youtube.com/@jayantdeshm

https://www.threads.net/@jayantdeshmukhofficial

https://x.com/jayantdeshm

Copyright @2024 Jayant Deshmukh

Prologue

The story of this book begins long before I sat down to write its first word. It began in the quiet observation of a world grappling with challenges too big to ignore. As someone who has spent 1 and half decade in digital transformation, often straddling the fascinating realms of technology and human needs, I found myself drawn increasingly toward one undeniable truth: **healthcare, the cornerstone of human well-being, was in desperate need of innovation.**

The seeds of this realization were planted during my travels and professional engagements across diverse geographies. From bustling metropolitan cities with cutting-edge hospitals to rural villages where medical facilities are scarce, the disparity in access to quality healthcare was stark. Yet, amidst this disparity, a common thread united them all: a system buckling under the weight of inefficiencies, rising costs, and unmet needs.

For centuries, medicine has relied on the brilliance of human minds and hands. From the time of Hippocrates, often called the Father of Medicine, to the revolutionary work of pioneers like Marie Curie and Alexander Fleming, advancements in healthcare were driven by sheer determination, curiosity, and the pursuit of knowledge. But as humanity entered the 21st century, it became evident that traditional approaches, no matter how brilliant, could not keep pace with the growing complexity of healthcare demands.

This is where **digital transformation** steps in—not as a replacement for human expertise but as its most powerful ally.

In 2020, the world faced one of its greatest modern health crises: the COVID-19 pandemic. It exposed the cracks in healthcare systems worldwide, from the inability to predict and manage outbreaks to the logistical challenges of distributing resources like vaccines and protective equipment. It was a turning point—a wake-up call for us all.

I vividly recall watching the chaos unfold. Patients overwhelmed hospitals, frontline workers were stretched to their limits, and communities struggled to stay connected amidst lockdowns. Yet, even in the darkest moments, there were glimmers of hope. Artificial intelligence (AI) tools were used to track the virus's spread, telemedicine brought doctors into patients' homes, and data analytics helped allocate resources more efficiently.

It became clear to me that this crisis was not just a challenge but an opportunity—a chance to reimagine healthcare through the lens of **technology-driven transformation**.

Digital transformation is not merely a trend; it's a **necessity** in medicine and healthcare. At its core, it is about harnessing the power of technology to solve real-world problems, improve efficiencies, and, most importantly, enhance the human experience.

Healthcare systems have historically been reactive, treating diseases as they occur. But with the advent of digital tools, we are witnessing a paradigm shift toward **proactive and preventive care**. For example:

- **Predictive analytics** is allowing us to foresee outbreaks of diseases before they happen.
- **Wearable devices** are helping individuals monitor their health in real time, catching warning signs early.

- **AI algorithms** are assisting doctors in diagnosing diseases with unparalleled accuracy, sometimes even better than the human eye.

This transformation extends beyond patient care to the very foundations of healthcare operations. Hospitals are now optimizing their resources, from scheduling staff to managing inventory, through data-driven insights. Supply chains are becoming smarter, ensuring that life-saving medicines and equipment are always available when and where they're needed.

Digital transformation is also democratizing healthcare. Technologies like **telemedicine** and **mobile health apps** are breaking down geographical barriers, bringing quality care to underserved regions.

As much as I am a believer in the power of technology, I am equally passionate about the **human stories** that drive it. Every breakthrough in digital healthcare is not just about the algorithms or devices; it's about the people whose lives are touched and transformed.

Take, for instance, the story of Ravi, a farmer from a remote village in India. Ravi's family had long suffered from limited access to healthcare. But one day, when his father began experiencing chest pains, a telemedicine service connected them to a cardiologist in a metropolitan city within minutes. Through a mobile ECG device powered by AI, the doctor diagnosed an impending heart attack and arranged for immediate intervention, saving his life.

Or consider Maria, a single mother in Brazil, managing her diabetes with the help of a smartphone app. The app monitors her blood sugar levels, reminds her to take her medication, and even suggests meal plans tailored to her condition. For Maria, this isn't just technology—it's a lifeline that helps her stay healthy for her children.

These are the stories that inspire me. They remind us that while technology may be the enabler, **human lives are the ultimate beneficiaries.**

As I worked on projects that spanned continents and industries, I often found myself drawn to the intersection of AI and healthcare. There was something profoundly satisfying about watching technology bridge the gap between unmet needs and innovative solutions.

One of the most memorable moments in my career was collaborating with a team to develop an AI tool for **early cancer detection.** The project involved integrating vast amounts of data—medical histories, genetic profiles, imaging scans—and training an algorithm to identify potential signs of cancer. The results were astounding: not only did the AI system improve detection rates, but it also gave doctors a tool that complemented their expertise rather than replacing it.

That project was a turning point for me. It solidified my belief that **AI and digital transformation** are not just about technology; they are about **partnerships**—between machines and humans, between innovators and caregivers, and between technology and society.

What This Book Offers You

This book is my attempt to distill years of experiences, observations, and lessons into a guide that is both **informative** and **inspiring.** It's for anyone who shares my passion for healthcare, whether you're a medical professional, a technologist, a policymaker, or simply someone curious about the future.

In the chapters ahead, you'll explore how AI is transforming every aspect of healthcare:

- From **diagnostics and drug discovery** to **patient engagement** and **global health challenges.**
- From **surgical precision** and **robotics** to **personalized wellness programs.**
- From the **ethical considerations** that guide us to the **inspiring stories** that remind us why this work matters.

Each chapter is infused with real-world examples, step-by-step insights, and a vision for what lies ahead.

As you embark on this journey, I invite you to see yourself as part of the story. The future of healthcare isn't just about what AI can do; it's about what **we all can do** together. Whether you're developing the next groundbreaking technology, advocating for fair policies, or simply making informed choices about your own health, your role is vital.

Together, we can create a world where healthcare is not just a privilege but a right—a world where technology serves humanity in its most profound sense.

This book is not just a roadmap; it's a **call to action.** Let's embrace this new dawn in medicine and healthcare, and let's shape it with wisdom, compassion, and a shared commitment to a healthier tomorrow.

Welcome to the journey. Let's begin.

Introduction

When I look back at my journey in artificial intelligence (AI) and global healthcare, I can't help but marvel at the incredible intersection of technology and human needs. My path has taken me through the bustling innovation hubs of Silicon Valley, the quiet determination of researchers in European labs, and the resilience of healthcare workers in underserved regions of Asia and Africa.

Each step along the way has reinforced a singular truth: **healthcare is not just about curing diseases—it's about empowering people to live healthier, fuller lives.** And AI, in its boundless potential, is emerging as one of the most transformative tools in this mission.

This book is not just a compendium of facts or theories. It is a culmination of experiences, observations, and aspirations—an attempt to bridge the often-intimidating world of AI with the deeply human realm of medicine.

A Personal Journey into AI and Global Healthcare

I have always been fascinated by technology and its ability to solve real-world problems. My early career revolved around implementing digital transformation strategies across industries. However, it wasn't until I began working on healthcare projects that I truly understood the transformative power of technology.

I remember one pivotal project with a healthcare provider in Southeast Asia. They were grappling with overcrowded hospitals, limited diagnostic tools, and an aging population with chronic diseases. It was a daunting challenge, but it was also an opportunity. We introduced an AI-based system that could analyze patient records, identify high-risk cases, and prioritize care. The results were nothing short of remarkable. Emergency room wait times dropped by 40%, doctors reported improved efficiency, and, most importantly, patients received better, faster care.

This was a turning point in my journey. It showed me that AI wasn't just about automation or data crunching—it was about **enhancing human capabilities** and ensuring that no one was left behind in their pursuit of health and well-being.

Over the years, my work has taken me to countries with vastly different healthcare landscapes. In India, I've seen AI-enabled telemedicine bring specialists into the homes of rural families. In Europe, I've witnessed AI tools assist surgeons in achieving precision previously unimaginable. In Africa, I've been inspired by grassroots innovations using AI to combat epidemics. Each encounter added another layer of understanding to my vision: that AI is not a luxury; it is a necessity for creating a healthier, more equitable world.

Why This Book?

The idea for this book came from a simple yet profound realization: **AI is reshaping healthcare, but its potential remains misunderstood or untapped by many.**

AI, to most people, still feels like science fiction. They hear about robots performing surgeries or algorithms predicting diseases, but the practical implications of these advancements often feel distant. Through this book, I aim to demystify AI, making it accessible to anyone curious about its role in healthcare.

The purpose of this book is threefold:

1. **To Educate:** I want to help readers understand the transformative potential of AI in healthcare, from improving diagnostics to enhancing patient experiences.
2. **To Inspire:** Through real-life examples and stories, I hope to showcase the human side of AI and how it is making a tangible difference in people's lives.
3. **To Empower:** Whether you're a healthcare professional, a policymaker, or a technology enthusiast, I want you to see your role in this journey and feel equipped to contribute to it.

This book is my way of bringing together the knowledge I've gained over the years and sharing it with a broader audience.

Technological Advancements in Healthcare: A New Era

The past decade has been a watershed moment for technology in healthcare. From wearable devices that track our every step to AI algorithms capable of diagnosing diseases with pinpoint accuracy, the innovations are staggering. But what's even more remarkable is the **potential** of these technologies to transform lives.

Let's start with diagnostics. In the past, detecting diseases like cancer often relied on invasive procedures or the trained eye of a specialist. Today, AI-powered tools can analyze medical images, identify anomalies, and provide diagnoses with incredible accuracy. For example, Google Health's AI system has shown promise in detecting breast cancer in mammograms more accurately than human radiologists. This isn't about replacing doctors; it's about giving them tools to be even better at what they do.

Then there's the revolution in drug discovery. Developing a new drug traditionally takes years, if not decades, and costs billions of dollars. AI is changing that. By analyzing vast datasets of medical research and patient information, AI can identify potential drug candidates in a fraction of the time. During the COVID-19 pandemic, AI tools played a crucial role in accelerating vaccine development.

But perhaps the most visible impact of AI is in patient care. Virtual health assistants, chatbots, and telemedicine platforms are making healthcare more accessible than ever. Take Babylon Health, a UK-based AI-powered platform that allows patients to consult doctors, check symptoms, and receive personalized health advice—all from the comfort of their homes.

These advancements are not just technological milestones; they are **human triumphs.** They represent our ability to leverage innovation for the greater good.

The Human Touch in Technology

As exciting as these innovations are, it's important to remember that technology alone is not the answer. At its core, healthcare is about **people**—patients, caregivers, doctors, and communities. AI's true power lies in its ability to complement human expertise and bridge gaps in care.

One of the most heartening examples of this is the use of AI in rural healthcare. In many parts of the world, access to specialists is limited. AI tools, combined with mobile technology, are helping to change that. For instance, in sub-Saharan Africa, AI-enabled ultrasound devices are empowering community health workers to perform prenatal scans and detect complications early. These tools don't replace doctors; they extend their reach, ensuring that no woman is left without care during her pregnancy.

Similarly, AI is helping to address health inequities. In the United States, algorithms are being used to identify social determinants of health—factors like housing, education, and income—that impact a person's well-being. By addressing these factors, healthcare providers can deliver more personalized and effective care.

A Glimpse into the Future

As we stand on the brink of a new era in healthcare, the possibilities are endless. Imagine a world where hospitals are fully connected ecosystems, where wearable devices alert us to health issues before they become critical, and where AI-powered tools help eradicate diseases that have plagued humanity for centuries.

But with these possibilities come challenges. Ethical considerations, data privacy, and the need for robust regulations are just a few of the hurdles we must navigate. This book doesn't shy away from these complexities. Instead, it seeks to explore them, providing a balanced view of both the opportunities and the responsibilities that come with AI-driven healthcare.

An Invitation to the Reader

This book is as much about you as it is about AI and healthcare. Whether you're a seasoned professional in the field, a curious learner, or someone who simply wants to understand how technology is shaping our lives, this journey is for you.

As you turn the pages, I invite you to see the stories behind the innovations—the patients whose lives have been saved, the doctors whose jobs have been made easier, and the communities that have been empowered.

Together, let's explore the boundless potential of AI in healthcare and imagine a future where technology and humanity work hand

Copyright @2024 Jayant Deshmukh

in hand to create a healthier, more connected world. Welcome to this transformative journey. Let's begin.

"The future of healthcare is not about machines replacing humans; it's about empowering humanity with technology to heal, connect, and transform lives."

– Jayant Deshmukh

Copyright @2024 Jayant Deshmukh

Chapter 1: The Current State of Healthcare and Medicine

Healthcare has been the cornerstone of human progress for centuries. Yet, in our modern world, the healthcare industry faces immense challenges—accessibility, affordability, quality, and efficiency. Despite the significant technological strides we've made in the last few decades, these issues continue to plague healthcare systems worldwide. In this chapter, we'll explore these challenges in-depth, how they affect millions of people, and how, with the right technologies and human ingenuity, we can overcome them.

The Challenges: A Global Perspective

I have had the privilege of traveling to various countries and working alongside healthcare professionals across different continents, which has provided me with a unique vantage point to understand the global healthcare system. While the challenges are many, some issues stand out clearly as barriers to effective healthcare. These challenges—access, affordability, quality, and efficiency—are interconnected, and their impact is far-reaching. Let's break them down one by one:

1. Access to Healthcare: The Ever-Present Barrier

One of the biggest challenges facing the global healthcare system today is access. In many parts of the world, access to quality healthcare is a privilege, not a right. There are rural and underserved areas where healthcare professionals are few and far between, and people have to travel long distances for even basic care. I've personally witnessed this in my travels across parts of Africa and Southeast Asia, where patients walked for hours to reach a healthcare facility, sometimes with limited resources and outdated equipment.

A poignant memory that comes to mind is my visit to a rural village in India, where healthcare was sparse, and people had to travel 30 kilometers just to see a doctor. In such areas, basic health check-ups were a luxury, and the concept of preventative care was almost non-existent. For these communities, healthcare is an emergency, not a continuous service.

The lack of infrastructure—especially in developing regions—makes it nearly impossible for people to receive the care they need when they need it. And even in developed nations, healthcare access can be a challenge for certain demographics, such as low-income families, the elderly, and people living in remote areas.

2. Affordability: The High Cost of Healthcare

In many parts of the world, even when people have access to healthcare, the cost is prohibitive. The price of medical services and prescription drugs continues to rise globally, creating a stark divide between those who can afford care and those who cannot.

During my time in the United States, I was struck by the rising costs of healthcare, particularly when speaking with families struggling to cover insurance premiums and co-pays for necessary treatments. A hospital visit in the U.S. can easily cost thousands of dollars, even for basic consultations. Many families face a choice between receiving life-saving care or going into debt.

In lower-income countries, the issue of affordability takes on a different form. For example, in some African nations, many people still rely on traditional medicine simply because they cannot afford even the most basic healthcare services. In these regions, the cost of even a basic check-up or medication can be an insurmountable barrier.

3. Quality: Ensuring Good Healthcare for All

The quality of healthcare varies drastically from one place to another. I've witnessed firsthand how healthcare quality can be compromised by factors such as a lack of trained professionals, inadequate medical equipment, and insufficient funding. In some parts of the world, the healthcare system is overburdened and under-resourced, leading to long waiting times, misdiagnoses, and even avoidable deaths.

While quality care is widely available in wealthy nations, it's a different story in poorer regions, where healthcare professionals often work in hospitals with outdated equipment. In rural hospitals, where I've worked alongside local doctors in East Africa, I've seen physicians diagnose and treat patients with limited tools and technology, often improvising in ways that would be unheard of in well-equipped hospitals.

But even in developed countries, issues with quality arise. One of the most common concerns is the overburdened healthcare system, where physicians see hundreds of patients in a day, leaving little time for personalized care. This shortage of time, combined with administrative burdens, has led to burnout among healthcare professionals, which in turn affects the overall quality of care.

4. Efficiency: Streamlining the System

Efficiency is perhaps one of the greatest hurdles in modern healthcare. As the global population continues to grow, so too does the demand for healthcare services. Hospitals and clinics are increasingly overwhelmed by patient loads, and healthcare professionals are stretched thin.

I recall working in the UK, where hospitals often faced difficulties in managing patient flows and timely appointments. One instance stands out: A hospital had to delay surgery for patients because of a backlog in pre-operative assessments. Such inefficiencies lead to delays in treatment, miscommunication, and overall frustration for patients.

Additionally, the vast amounts of data generated by healthcare systems are often poorly managed. Many hospitals still rely on paper records, leading to issues with data accuracy and sharing. Patients frequently have to repeat their medical history multiple times because the information isn't readily available to the healthcare provider, wasting time and creating inefficiencies.

Key Differences in Healthcare Systems Worldwide

In my travels, I have had the privilege of experiencing different healthcare systems, from the public health systems of Europe to the private healthcare models in the United States, and the community-focused healthcare in Southeast Asia. Each system has its strengths and weaknesses, and understanding these differences provides insight into how we might improve global healthcare.

1. The Public Healthcare System (Europe)

In countries like the UK, Germany, and France, public healthcare systems aim to provide universal coverage. These countries have a strong social safety net for healthcare, where everyone, regardless of income, can access basic services. However, the challenge often lies in long wait times and overburdened facilities. While these systems are highly efficient in many ways, they face increasing pressure due to aging populations and the rising cost of healthcare.

2. The Private Healthcare System (United States)

The United States' healthcare system is heavily privatized, with a mix of public and private insurance options. While patients in the U.S. have access to cutting-edge medical technology and treatments, affordability remains a significant issue, particularly for those without insurance or with insufficient coverage. Healthcare costs continue to rise, leading to disparities between wealthy and low-income patients.

3. The Hybrid Model (India, South Africa, Brazil)

In many developing nations, including India and South Africa, there's a hybrid model of healthcare that combines public and private sectors. While public healthcare provides basic services, private healthcare offers higher-quality services at a premium cost. However, even in the private sector, resources can be limited, and in rural areas, access to specialized treatments is often restricted.

I saw firsthand in India how patients in rural villages had limited access to quality healthcare. However, in urban centers, private healthcare was of an international standard, but only a select few could afford it.

Technology: The Catalyst for Change

Despite these challenges, technology has already begun reshaping the healthcare industry in profound ways. As I've seen across different nations, from the bustling cities of North America to the more remote areas of Africa and Asia, one thing is clear: technology is key to overcoming these barriers.

1. Telemedicine: Bridging the Gap

Telemedicine is one of the most exciting innovations that have the potential to address the accessibility problem. During my time working in rural Africa, I witnessed telemedicine's ability to connect remote areas with specialized doctors. Patients could consult with doctors thousands of miles away, receiving expert advice and treatment recommendations via video consultations. This technology has been instrumental in breaking down geographical barriers and providing essential healthcare to underserved populations.

In developed countries, telemedicine has become a vital tool during the COVID-19 pandemic, enabling doctors to continue treating patients remotely. In India, where I've spent considerable time working with healthcare startups, telemedicine has been integrated into primary care, allowing doctors to monitor patients in rural areas through mobile apps.

2. Electronic Health Records (EHR): Improving Efficiency and Quality

Electronic Health Records (EHR) have been pivotal in improving healthcare efficiency and quality. Gone are the days of paper-based records, where patient information was often incomplete or inaccessible. EHR systems ensure that patient information is stored securely and can be shared between healthcare providers seamlessly.

In countries like the UK and the US, EHR has greatly improved the coordination of care. I've worked with hospitals that have integrated EHR systems, where a doctor can access a patient's entire medical history with just a few clicks. This not only saves time but also prevents errors that could arise from inaccurate or missing records.

Conclusion: A New Era of Healthcare

As we move forward, the role of technology in healthcare will only grow. AI, machine learning, and telemedicine are just the beginning. I believe that with the right combination of technology, policy changes, and global collaboration, we can overcome the healthcare challenges that exist today.

Through my journey, I have witnessed the transformative power of technology in healthcare. The dream of accessible, affordable, high-quality, and efficient healthcare for all is within our reach. But it will take collective action, continued innovation, and a commitment to making healthcare a right, not a privilege, for all.

In the following chapters, we'll dive deeper into how AI, in particular, is poised to drive the next phase of healthcare transformation.

Chapter 2: Demystifying Artificial Intelligence in Healthcare

Artificial Intelligence (AI) is a word that has become synonymous with innovation and transformation. When we think about AI, images of futuristic robots or self-driving cars might come to mind. However, what many people don't realize is that AI is already making a huge impact in healthcare today, transforming the way doctors diagnose diseases, treat patients, and manage healthcare systems.

As someone who has spent years studying AI and its application across industries, I've had the privilege of seeing AI's impact on healthcare firsthand. I've worked with hospitals in different parts of the world, from high-tech institutions in the United States to rural healthcare facilities in Africa, and have seen AI evolve into one of the most powerful tools for medical professionals. In this chapter, we'll simplify what AI is, the technologies behind it, and how it is already shaping the future of healthcare.

The Fundamentals of AI in Healthcare

Let's start by breaking down what AI really is, in simple terms. At its core, **Artificial Intelligence** refers to the simulation of human intelligence in machines—machines that can think, learn, and make decisions. Imagine a system that can read medical records, recognize patterns in data, and make recommendations based on the information it processes. That's AI at work.

AI in healthcare is not just about machines replacing doctors. It's about augmenting the skills of healthcare professionals by providing them with tools that make their work faster, more accurate, and more efficient. AI is here to support doctors, nurses, and healthcare workers, allowing them to make better decisions, faster.

For example, when a doctor is looking at a chest X-ray to diagnose lung cancer, AI-powered software can analyze that image in seconds, highlighting areas of concern that the doctor may have missed. This way, AI helps the doctor make more accurate diagnoses, improving patient outcomes.

I've been fortunate enough to witness this firsthand. A few years ago, I visited a hospital in the US where AI technology had been integrated into the diagnostic process. The radiologists I spoke to were enthusiastic about the support AI provided. They explained that AI helped them detect anomalies much faster, giving them more time to focus on treating patients.

But the question many ask is: **How does AI do all of this?** Let's dive into the key technologies that power AI in healthcare.

Key Technologies Powering AI in Healthcare

To understand how AI works in healthcare, we need to explore the technologies behind it. The main technologies driving AI include **Machine Learning (ML)**, **Natural Language Processing (NLP)**, **Computer Vision**, and **Robotics**. These technologies are at the heart of many AI applications, and each plays a critical role in transforming healthcare systems.

1. Machine Learning (ML)

Machine Learning is a subset of AI that allows systems to learn from data and improve over time, without being explicitly programmed. Think of it like teaching a child how to recognize animals. You show the child many pictures of cats and dogs, and after a while, they start to distinguish between the two. ML works in a similar way, where an algorithm is trained using large amounts of data and learns to make predictions or decisions based on that data.

In healthcare, ML is used to predict patient outcomes, detect diseases early, and recommend treatments. For example, a machine learning model can be trained on thousands of medical records to identify patterns that could indicate a higher risk of heart disease. These patterns could be things like a history of smoking, high blood pressure, or high cholesterol. The system can then alert the doctor to a patient's risk, allowing for early intervention.

I remember a visit to a hospital in the UK, where ML algorithms were used to predict the likelihood of patients developing diabetes. The system analyzed thousands of patient records and flagged individuals at high risk, allowing doctors to provide targeted interventions before the disease developed. This kind of predictive power is changing the way healthcare professionals approach preventive care.

2. Natural Language Processing (NLP)

Natural Language Processing is another powerful AI technology that focuses on understanding and processing human language. In healthcare, this means interpreting medical records, doctor-patient conversations, and research papers. NLP helps AI systems "understand" text and speech, making it possible for healthcare professionals to access relevant information quickly and efficiently.

A good example of NLP in action is in **clinical documentation**. Doctors and nurses spend a significant amount of time documenting patient information in electronic health records (EHRs). But with NLP, AI can analyze patient notes, extract important information, and even suggest next steps based on the medical history of the patient. This helps reduce the time healthcare professionals spend on administrative tasks and allows them to focus more on patient care.

During a project I worked on in India, NLP was used to analyze patient feedback and reports in real-time, helping doctors better understand the concerns of their patients and adjust treatments accordingly. NLP also enabled the system to recommend the best treatment options based on previous cases with similar symptoms, vastly improving decision-making.

3. Computer Vision

Computer Vision is an AI technology that allows computers to interpret and understand visual information from the world, such as images and videos. In healthcare, computer vision is primarily used in medical imaging, such as X-rays, CT scans, and MRIs, where the system can "see" and analyze medical images to help doctors make diagnoses.

Take radiology, for example. One of the most promising applications of computer vision in healthcare is the ability of AI to analyze radiological images. Computer vision algorithms can examine X-rays for signs of pneumonia, cancer, or fractures, identifying potential issues that may be difficult for human eyes to spot. These algorithms are often more accurate than the human eye, particularly in identifying subtle abnormalities.

I've worked with several hospitals where computer vision was used to assist doctors in diagnosing cancer. One example was a partnership with a hospital in Singapore, where an AI system was trained to recognize early signs of lung cancer on chest X-rays. The results were remarkable—AI helped identify tumors that were missed by radiologists, leading to early detection and improved survival rates.

4. Robotics

In the world of healthcare, robots have come a long way from the science fiction movies. Today, robots are used in surgeries, rehabilitation, and even patient care. These robots are powered by AI algorithms that allow them to perform tasks with precision and accuracy, often in ways that would be impossible for humans.

One of the most exciting applications of robotics is in **robotic surgery**. Robots, guided by AI, can assist surgeons in performing complex procedures with greater precision. This not only reduces the risk of complications but also leads to quicker recovery times for patients. In my travels, I've had the chance to observe robotic surgeries, and I can tell you that the precision with which these machines operate is truly astonishing.

In the US, a well-known robot named **da Vinci** is used for minimally invasive surgeries. With da Vinci, surgeons can perform delicate procedures through tiny incisions, using robotic arms that offer far more dexterity than human hands. The AI behind the system analyzes the patient's anatomy and provides real-time feedback to the surgeon, making surgeries faster and more accurate.

Real-World Examples of AI's Applications in Healthcare

Now that we understand the key technologies behind AI, let's take a look at how they are being applied in real-world healthcare settings.

1. Early Diagnosis of Diseases

One of the most powerful applications of AI in healthcare is early diagnosis. Early detection of diseases like cancer, diabetes, and heart disease can save lives. AI systems can analyze patient data, medical images, and even genetic information to identify early signs of disease long before symptoms appear.

For example, in the UK, an AI system called **DeepMind** developed by Google has been used to detect eye diseases by analyzing retinal scans. The AI system can identify conditions like diabetic retinopathy and age-related macular degeneration, diseases that can lead to blindness if not caught early. In many cases, the AI was able to detect these diseases earlier than human doctors could, giving patients a better chance at successful treatment.

Similarly, AI is being used to detect **breast cancer** in mammograms. Researchers have developed machine learning models that can analyze mammogram images with an accuracy level comparable to experienced radiologists. In a study conducted at a hospital in the US, AI algorithms were able to identify breast cancer with 94% accuracy, reducing the likelihood of misdiagnoses.

2. Personalized Treatment Plans

AI is also making waves in the field of **personalized medicine**, where treatment plans are tailored to the individual's unique genetic makeup and medical history. By analyzing vast amounts of patient data, AI can recommend the most effective treatments for a patient based on their specific condition.

A great example of this is the use of AI in **oncology**, where AI models analyze cancer patients' genetic data to recommend personalized treatment options. In one instance, an AI system was used to analyze genetic mutations in a cancer patient's tumor and then recommended a targeted therapy that had never been considered before. The treatment proved to be successful, demonstrating how AI can improve the effectiveness of personalized treatment.

3. AI in Drug Discovery

The process of discovering new drugs is long, costly, and fraught with uncertainty. But AI is revolutionizing this process by helping researchers identify promising drug candidates faster and more accurately. AI algorithms analyze chemical compounds, predicting which ones will have the desired effect on the body. This can drastically speed up the process of drug development, potentially saving billions of dollars and years of research.

For instance, **Atomwise**, an AI-powered platform, uses machine learning to predict the effectiveness of various chemical compounds in treating diseases like Ebola and cancer. In collaboration with researchers, Atomwise was able to identify a compound that could help fight the Ebola virus, which led to a faster drug development process.

Conclusion: The Future of AI in Healthcare

As we look to the future, it's clear that AI will play an increasingly important role in healthcare. It will help doctors diagnose diseases earlier, provide personalized treatments, and improve the overall efficiency of healthcare systems. AI is not here to replace doctors; it's here to empower them to do their jobs better and faster.

The potential of AI in healthcare is limitless, and as the technology continues to evolve, we can expect even more breakthroughs. For those of us who work in the field of AI, there's an exciting road ahead as we explore new ways to integrate these technologies into healthcare systems around the world. And as we continue to innovate, the ultimate goal remains the same: to improve the health and well-being of people around the world.

This is just the beginning of the AI revolution in healthcare. The possibilities are endless, and the impact will be felt for generations to come.

Chapter 3: AI in Diagnostics and Imaging

The power of **Artificial Intelligence** (AI) to transform the healthcare landscape has already begun to unfold, and one of the most exciting areas where we see this transformation is in **diagnostics and medical imaging**. Imagine a world where diseases like cancer, heart conditions, and rare illnesses can be detected with unparalleled speed and accuracy. A world where AI is not just a tool for doctors, but a trusted assistant—one that assists in interpreting medical images, analyzing patient data, and ultimately improving the precision of diagnoses.

In this chapter, I will take you on a journey through the incredible advancements AI is bringing to the field of **medical imaging**. We will explore how AI is playing a critical role in analyzing complex medical images, including **radiology**, **pathology**, and **dermatology**. Together, we will look at real-world examples, where AI is making remarkable strides in early disease detection, personalized medicine, and diagnosing conditions that are often too complex or rare for the human eye to catch.

Let me share with you a story from one of my trips to a hospital in a small town. The hospital had limited access to the resources we often take for granted in larger cities. However, they had just integrated AI-based imaging tools to assist their doctors. The team there was excited, but skeptical. They were unsure how an AI system could enhance their work. But once they began using the AI tools, everything changed. The accuracy of diagnoses improved significantly, and patients received the right treatments much faster than before.

This story is just one of many that I've encountered during my travels. AI in diagnostics is not just about improving accuracy—

it's about giving healthcare providers the ability to act swiftly and intelligently, improving patient outcomes and reducing unnecessary costs. Now, let's dive into how AI is revolutionizing diagnostics and medical imaging.

AI's Role in Analyzing Medical Imaging

Medical imaging plays a pivotal role in diagnosing and treating diseases. For decades, doctors have relied on **X-rays, CT scans, MRIs, ultrasound images**, and **pathological slides** to identify and monitor diseases. These images are crucial in diagnosing conditions ranging from broken bones to tumors, infections, and cardiovascular problems.

Traditionally, doctors and radiologists would manually review these images to identify abnormalities. However, this process can be time-consuming and subject to human error. Now, with the advent of AI technologies, the analysis of medical imaging has taken a giant leap forward. AI algorithms, particularly **computer vision** technologies, are being integrated into imaging software, enabling machines to "see" and interpret medical images as a human would, but with far greater precision and speed.

AI systems are trained using millions of annotated images, learning to identify patterns, shapes, and features that may indicate the presence of a disease. The power of AI lies in its ability to identify even the smallest nuances that might be overlooked by the human eye, and it does this in a fraction of the time.

Take, for example, the case of **radiology**—a field where AI is already showing remarkable success. Radiologists use X-rays, CT scans, and MRIs to detect a wide range of conditions, from fractures to cancerous tumors. AI can help detect early signs of diseases like **lung cancer, breast cancer, brain tumors**, and **heart disease** by analyzing images much faster and more accurately than a human could.

In one such example, a group of researchers in the U.S. used an AI algorithm to analyze mammograms and identify early signs of breast cancer. The results were astounding. The AI system not only detected the presence of cancer with remarkable accuracy but also identified tumors that radiologists had missed. This example highlights how AI can help catch diseases early, leading to better outcomes for patients.

Another incredible breakthrough involves **pathology**, which is the study of tissue samples. In the past, pathologists had to manually examine slides of tissue samples under a microscope to diagnose diseases such as cancer. AI is changing this by analyzing digital pathology slides with great precision. With the help of deep learning algorithms, AI can identify patterns in tissue samples, detect cancerous cells, and even determine the type and stage of cancer, all in a fraction of the time it would take a pathologist to do so manually.

Case Studies: AI Detecting Cancer, Heart Diseases, and Rare Conditions

One of the most powerful applications of AI in diagnostics is its ability to detect **cancer** early—often at stages when treatment options are most effective. Let's look at some real-life examples that illustrate the incredible potential of AI in detecting cancer, heart disease, and rare conditions.

1. AI in Detecting Cancer

Cancer is one of the deadliest diseases in the world, and early detection is crucial in improving survival rates. In recent years, AI has become a vital tool in identifying cancer at an earlier stage, which increases the chances of successful treatment.

Let's consider **AI in detecting lung cancer**, one of the deadliest cancers worldwide. A team of researchers in the UK developed an AI algorithm that analyzed CT scans of patients to identify signs of lung cancer. What makes this technology so impressive is the algorithm's ability to identify very small lesions, even in early stages, that radiologists often missed.

The AI system used **deep learning**, a subset of machine learning, to learn from thousands of CT scans and recognize patterns indicative of lung cancer. When tested on new scans, the system identified 94% of the cases of lung cancer, outperforming human radiologists in terms of accuracy. This breakthrough is revolutionary in the fight against lung cancer, as it enables doctors to detect the disease at its earliest, most treatable stages.

Another AI success story comes from **breast cancer detection**. AI-powered systems are being used to analyze mammograms with much higher accuracy than human radiologists. One such system, developed by Google's DeepMind, was tested against a group of radiologists in the UK and the U.S. It was found to be better at detecting breast cancer than the radiologists, with fewer false positives and negatives. This breakthrough could drastically reduce the need for unnecessary biopsies and lead to earlier, more accurate diagnoses.

2. AI in Detecting Heart Diseases

Heart disease is another area where AI is making a significant impact. Cardiologists use medical imaging to assess the condition of the heart, but analyzing these images can be time-consuming and requires years of expertise. AI is streamlining this process, making it faster and more accurate.

For example, AI algorithms are now being used to analyze **echocardiograms** (ultrasound images of the heart). These algorithms can quickly assess heart function, including detecting signs of **heart failure, arrhythmias**, or **valvular diseases**. In one study, an AI system was trained on over 30,000 echocardiograms to identify potential heart issues. The system outperformed human cardiologists in detecting heart conditions, including early signs of heart failure that might otherwise have been missed.

Moreover, AI is also helping detect **coronary artery disease (CAD)**, which can lead to heart attacks. In one example, AI was used to analyze **coronary CT angiography** images to detect blockages in the arteries. The AI system identified patients at high risk of CAD with high accuracy, helping doctors intervene early and reduce the risk of heart attacks.

3. AI in Diagnosing Rare Conditions

AI is also making waves in diagnosing **rare diseases**, which often present challenges for doctors due to their complexity and rarity. One notable example is the use of AI in diagnosing **rare genetic disorders**. Geneticists often rely on medical imaging, clinical data, and family history to diagnose such conditions, but this can take years and result in misdiagnoses.

In a case study from a hospital in Canada, an AI-powered system was developed to analyze **genetic data** to help doctors diagnose rare genetic conditions like **muscular dystrophy** and **sickle cell anemia**. The AI system used **machine learning algorithms** to compare the patient's genetic data with a vast database of known genetic disorders, accurately predicting the likelihood of specific rare conditions. This technology is a game-changer, allowing doctors to provide earlier diagnoses and more effective treatments for rare diseases.

AI-Driven Precision Diagnostics and its Role in Personalized Medicine

As we move towards the future, one of the most exciting applications of AI in healthcare is its role in **precision diagnostics** and **personalized medicine**. Precision diagnostics is all about tailoring healthcare to the individual, based on their unique genetic makeup, environment, and lifestyle.

AI is playing a crucial role in this personalized approach by analyzing **genomic data, medical histories**, and **lifestyle factors** to predict diseases, recommend personalized treatment plans, and optimize healthcare outcomes. For example, AI can analyze a patient's genetic data to determine the best course of treatment for conditions like cancer. Based on the genetic mutations present in the tumor, AI can suggest the most effective targeted therapies, which have a much higher success rate compared to traditional treatments.

This is particularly valuable in **oncology**, where each patient's cancer may behave differently depending on their genetic makeup. AI is enabling doctors to make more accurate decisions about the type of treatment that will work best for each individual, ensuring that patients receive the most effective care.

Additionally, AI is being used to predict **drug responses** in patients, helping doctors identify which medications are likely to be most effective, based on a patient's specific genetic profile. This is a major step forward in reducing the trial-and-error approach that often accompanies traditional medicine.

In my experience, I've seen AI empower doctors to make decisions that are highly personalized, considering a patient's unique condition rather than relying on generalized treatments. For example, an AI system could analyze a patient's data and predict their likelihood of responding to a particular drug, significantly improving treatment outcomes and reducing unnecessary side effects.

Conclusion: The Promise of AI in Diagnostics and Imaging

AI is undoubtedly transforming diagnostics and medical imaging in ways we could only dream of a few decades ago. From detecting cancer early to diagnosing heart disease with greater precision, AI is enabling healthcare professionals to deliver faster, more accurate diagnoses. The integration of AI into medical imaging is revolutionizing the way doctors and specialists interpret complex data, providing them with the tools to make better decisions and ultimately improve patient outcomes.

But the story doesn't end there. AI is also driving us towards a future where **precision medicine** is the norm, not the exception. With AI, we are moving towards a world where healthcare is more personalized, more efficient, and more effective—where technology helps doctors make better decisions, and patients receive the best possible care.

As AI continues to evolve, the possibilities are endless. What excites me most is that we are only scratching the surface of what's possible. AI in diagnostics and medical imaging has the potential to change not just how we diagnose and treat diseases but also how we approach healthcare as a whole.

Chapter 4: AI in Drug Discovery and Development

Imagine a world where a life-saving drug that could treat a deadly disease is discovered not in a matter of years, but in mere months. A world where AI accelerates the painstaking process of **drug discovery** and **development**, reducing the time and cost it takes to bring new medicines to market. We've heard about the challenges the pharmaceutical industry faces in bringing drugs to market—expensive, time-consuming, and fraught with risk. But with **Artificial Intelligence (AI)** now playing an increasingly pivotal role in this area, these challenges are becoming more surmountable. We're standing at the threshold of a new era in which AI is revolutionizing the way drugs are discovered, developed, and tested.

Let me take you through this exciting journey of AI in the **drug discovery** and **development** process, showing how it's not just improving efficiency but also driving us toward a future where new therapies are developed faster, more effectively, and more affordably.

A few years ago, I had the opportunity to visit a pharmaceutical research lab in a bustling city. The scientists there were incredibly passionate about discovering new drugs, but they were frustrated by the barriers in their path. Drug discovery was slow, with most projects taking **10 to 15 years** to complete and often costing billions of dollars. But one day, they began integrating AI into their workflow. That's when everything started to change.

AI allowed these researchers to simulate chemical reactions, analyze patterns in biological data, and sift through massive datasets of existing drugs and disease information at lightning speed. What used to take months or even years, they could now complete in days. The entire landscape of drug discovery began to change. From the initial concept of identifying potential drug candidates to clinical trials, AI was facilitating every step, making the process far more efficient and effective. The pace at which breakthroughs were happening left everyone in awe.

In this chapter, we'll dive deep into how AI accelerates drug discovery through simulations and pattern analysis, how it dramatically reduces costs and timelines, and how AI-powered clinical trials are improving participant selection and monitoring outcomes. By the end of this journey, you'll understand how AI is making a significant impact on the pharmaceutical industry, ultimately helping to save lives and improve health outcomes around the world.

How AI Accelerates Drug Discovery Through Simulations and Pattern Analysis

The process of **drug discovery** is a monumental challenge. Scientists must sift through millions of compounds, study their effects on the human body, and analyze how they interact with biological targets—proteins, enzymes, receptors, and genes. This process can take years, and there's no guarantee of success. Drug development is often like searching for a needle in a haystack, where most of the attempts fail, and only a small fraction of compounds ever make it to clinical trials.

This is where **AI** comes in to change the game. One of AI's most powerful capabilities lies in its ability to **simulate** complex biological processes and analyze patterns in vast datasets. AI algorithms are designed to learn from data, uncover hidden patterns, and predict outcomes based on past experiences. This is particularly valuable in drug discovery, where the complexity of biological systems means that a straightforward approach often falls short.

1. Drug Screening and Molecular Simulation

Imagine a traditional drug discovery process: researchers have to manually screen thousands of molecules to see if they bind to a specific protein that could be targeted to treat a disease. This process is labor-intensive and time-consuming. However, with AI, we now have **machine learning** models that can predict the properties of molecules with remarkable accuracy.

AI can simulate how different compounds interact with proteins, using **virtual screening** to predict which molecules are most likely to have a desired therapeutic effect. By leveraging **deep learning** and **neural networks**, AI systems analyze chemical structures to determine how molecules will behave. This allows scientists to focus on the most promising candidates for further testing, effectively narrowing down the number of compounds to test and speeding up the process.

One real-life example is how **Insilico Medicine**, an AI-driven biotechnology company, used AI to design a **novel drug** for **fibrosis**—a condition that causes scarring of organs. Using machine learning algorithms, they were able to identify potential drug candidates in just **46 days**, a process that traditionally takes years. By training the AI model on large datasets of molecular structures and biological outcomes, they found compounds that would have been impossible to identify using traditional methods.

2. Identifying New Drug Targets

One of the challenges in drug discovery is identifying which proteins or genes should be targeted for therapeutic purposes. AI plays a crucial role here by analyzing biological data to identify potential **drug targets** more accurately than traditional methods.

This process involves feeding AI algorithms with vast amounts of biological data—from genetic information to protein structures—and allowing the AI system to detect patterns that suggest which targets are most likely to yield effective therapies.

For instance, **AI-based platforms like Atomwise** analyze large biological datasets to predict which compounds might bind to a given target protein. This has proven to be particularly effective in identifying potential **antiviral drugs**. AI-powered drug design has already led to the discovery of compounds that could potentially fight against diseases like **Ebola** and **Zika virus**.

In the case of **cancer**, AI is helping scientists discover novel targets for therapies. AI algorithms analyze vast datasets of patient records, genetic mutations, and existing drugs to uncover hidden patterns that suggest new targets for cancer treatment. This has led to the development of **targeted therapies** that are designed to work more effectively for specific cancer types, based on the molecular profile of a patient's cancer cells.

Reducing Costs and Timelines for Developing Life-Saving Drugs

As I mentioned earlier, the traditional drug development process is expensive, time-consuming, and fraught with risk. It's a **$2.6 billion** gamble to bring a new drug to market, with most projects failing at some point during the long journey. The timeline for drug development can stretch to **15 years**, and there's no guarantee that a successful drug will emerge at the end.

AI is helping to **reduce costs** and **accelerate timelines** in several ways. First, by streamlining the early stages of drug discovery—such as molecule screening and target identification—AI helps pharmaceutical companies identify promising compounds and drug targets much more quickly. Instead of spending years in a trial-and-error process, AI allows researchers to focus on the most promising drug candidates, dramatically cutting down the time it takes to move forward.

AI also helps reduce costs by minimizing the need for large-scale laboratory experiments and human intervention. With AI simulations, researchers can predict how a drug will interact in the human body before they start testing it in real clinical settings. These simulations enable scientists to focus on drugs that are more likely to succeed, saving significant resources that would have been spent on failed experiments.

One incredible example of AI cutting down both cost and time is **Exscientia**, an AI-powered drug discovery company. They developed a novel **targeted cancer drug** in less than **12 months**, a process that would typically take years. The AI system was able to analyze vast datasets, simulate molecular interactions, and predict which compounds would work best, all while cutting costs by over **70%**.

Moreover, AI can help predict and analyze **side effects** and **toxicity** of drugs earlier in the process, further reducing the need for costly and lengthy clinical testing. In some cases, AI can even identify **repurposed drugs**—existing drugs that could be effective against new diseases. This process, known as **drug repurposing**, can save years and millions of dollars by using drugs that are already approved for other conditions.

AI-Powered Clinical Trials: Improving Participant Selection and Monitoring Outcomes

Once a promising drug candidate has been identified, it enters the clinical trial phase, where it is tested on human participants.

Clinical trials are essential for proving the safety and efficacy of a drug, but they are notoriously complex, expensive, and time-consuming. Recruiting the right participants, monitoring their progress, and analyzing trial results can take months or even years.

AI is revolutionizing the clinical trial process by improving **participant selection**, optimizing **trial design**, and enhancing **monitoring**. Here's how:

1. Improved Participant Selection

Selecting the right participants for clinical trials is a critical step in ensuring that the results are meaningful. Traditionally, participant selection was based on broad inclusion criteria, which sometimes led to **inconsistent results**. However, with AI, clinical trials can now be more **personalized**. AI analyzes patient data, such as **genetic profiles, medical histories**, and **lifestyle factors**, to select participants who are most likely to benefit from the drug being tested.

For example, AI algorithms can sift through electronic health records (EHR) to identify individuals with specific genetic mutations or conditions that are relevant to the drug being tested. This ensures that the clinical trial is focused on the right participants, improving the chances of success. In a study conducted by **Bristol Myers Squibb**, AI was used to identify patients who were most likely to respond to an experimental cancer treatment, significantly improving trial outcomes.

2. Enhanced Monitoring and Data Analysis

During clinical trials, monitoring patient progress is crucial to ensuring the drug is safe and effective. AI can assist in continuously analyzing patient data in real-time, looking for signs of adverse reactions, and adjusting treatment protocols as needed. AI systems can also analyze large amounts of data from wearable devices, such as heart rate monitors or glucose trackers, to track the patient's health throughout the trial.

For instance, AI-driven platforms are now being used to analyze data from **smart wearables** during clinical trials for heart disease medications. These devices continuously track vital signs like blood pressure, heart rate, and oxygen levels, which can be analyzed by AI to predict potential risks or side effects before they become serious. This level of real-time monitoring is invaluable in ensuring patient safety and improving the trial's overall success rate.

3. Predicting Trial Outcomes

One of the most powerful applications of AI in clinical trials is its ability to predict trial outcomes based on early data. Machine learning models can analyze data from ongoing trials and predict how different treatments will affect different patient populations. By identifying **patterns** in the data, AI can help researchers adjust the trial design to optimize success, leading to more accurate and quicker results.

In conclusion, AI is dramatically reshaping the landscape of drug discovery and development. From accelerating the discovery of new compounds to improving clinical trial outcomes, AI is enabling the pharmaceutical industry to create life-saving drugs faster, more efficiently, and more affordably. This transformation is not just improving the drug development process but is also paving the way for **personalized medicine**, where treatments are tailored to the unique genetic makeup and health profile of each patient.

The future of healthcare is brighter than ever before, and AI is at the heart of this revolution. As we continue to embrace AI in drug discovery, we are opening the door to new treatments, better outcomes, and a healthier world for all.

Copyright @2024 Jayant Deshmukh

Chapter 5: AI in Personalized Medicine

Imagine a world where each treatment you receive is custom-designed just for you—a treatment that takes into account not only your illness but also your unique genetic makeup, lifestyle, and environment. It sounds like something from a science fiction movie, but this is the reality that **personalized medicine**, powered by **Artificial Intelligence (AI)**, is bringing closer every day. AI is reshaping the healthcare landscape by allowing doctors to offer more **precise, effective,** and **tailored treatments** based on an individual's unique characteristics, rather than using the traditional one-size-fits-all approach.

I recall a moment from my travels when I visited a cutting-edge oncology center in a bustling city. The doctor there explained how they were using AI to treat cancer patients in ways never before imagined. The treatment was personalized—not just based on the patient's cancer type but also on their genetic profile, lifestyle choices, and even their environment. It was as if the treatment was designed for that individual's body, targeting the disease with the utmost precision while minimizing side effects. This experience made me realize that **personalized medicine**, which was once a dream, is fast becoming a reality.

In this chapter, we will delve into the world of **AI in personalized medicine**—how it tailors treatments based on a patient's genetic, environmental, and lifestyle factors. We'll explore how **AI and genomics** are working together to decode DNA and develop customized therapies. Finally, we will discuss real-world applications of AI in various medical fields, such as **oncology**, **cardiology**, and **rare diseases**, and how this innovation is transforming the way doctors approach treatment.

Tailoring Treatments Based on Genetic, Environmental, and Lifestyle Factors

Let's start by imagining a scenario in which your doctor is not just considering your symptoms but also your **genetic history, environmental exposures,** and **lifestyle choices** when determining the best course of treatment. The idea behind **personalized medicine** is that treatments should be tailored to the individual—recognizing that no two people are exactly alike, not even if they have the same disease. A person's **genetic makeup, lifestyle,** and **environment** all play significant roles in how they respond to certain treatments.

Traditionally, medicine has followed a **universal approach**, where the same treatment is often prescribed to all patients with the same disease, regardless of their unique characteristics. While this may work for some, it fails for many others. For example, **chemotherapy**, a common treatment for cancer, doesn't work the same way for every patient. It may work wonders for some but leave others with devastating side effects and minimal improvement.

With **AI**, we now have the ability to consider all of these factors to create a treatment plan that is personalized for each individual.

Genetic Factors

The first and most profound factor that AI takes into account is a patient's **genetic makeup**. Every individual's **DNA** is unique, and genetic variations can significantly affect how a person responds to medications. AI, combined with **genomic sequencing**, allows doctors to decode a patient's DNA and identify genetic mutations that could influence the effectiveness of a treatment. These insights enable healthcare providers to

tailor therapies that work with the body's natural biology rather than against it.

For instance, consider the case of **pharmacogenomics**, a field of personalized medicine that focuses on how a person's genetic makeup affects their response to drugs. AI models are now able to analyze genetic data to predict how a patient will respond to specific drugs, potentially preventing adverse reactions or ineffective treatments. Imagine a scenario where a patient is prescribed a drug, only for it to cause severe side effects. With AI analyzing their genetic data beforehand, this risk could be predicted and avoided.

One real-world example of this is the use of AI to guide **cancer treatments**. AI algorithms can analyze a patient's genetic profile, looking for specific mutations that may respond better to targeted therapies, such as **immunotherapy** or **targeted chemotherapy**, rather than traditional chemotherapy. For example, **HER2-positive breast cancer** patients benefit from a targeted therapy called **Herceptin**. AI helps to identify patients who will benefit most from this treatment by analyzing their genetic markers.

Environmental Factors

Beyond genetics, AI also considers **environmental factors** that play a crucial role in health outcomes. Factors like **exposure to toxins, pollution, diet, geography**, and even **stress levels** can all influence a person's susceptibility to disease and how they respond to treatment.

One example I encountered during my travels was in an urban center where the pollution levels were high, and respiratory diseases were common. AI was used to analyze environmental factors—like pollution levels in the air—along with individual patient data to predict who would be at greater risk of complications from diseases like **asthma** or **chronic obstructive pulmonary disease (COPD)**. AI could even suggest personalized treatment plans that accounted for these environmental triggers, helping patients avoid flare-ups and manage their conditions more effectively.

Lifestyle Factors

Another important element in personalized medicine is the consideration of **lifestyle factors**, such as **diet, exercise, sleep patterns**, and **stress levels**. AI, combined with data from **wearable devices**, allows doctors to get a real-time understanding of how these factors impact a patient's health and treatment. For example, AI can analyze data from fitness trackers, sleep monitors, and even mobile apps that track food intake to better understand a patient's habits and how these habits might influence their condition.

Imagine an AI system that integrates data from a patient's **diet** and **exercise regimen** to help manage **diabetes**. If a patient's blood sugar levels are high, AI can analyze their eating habits and activity levels to suggest more personalized lifestyle changes or adjustments to their medication. This level of personalization ensures that patients receive the most effective and sustainable treatment possible.

AI and Genomics: Decoding DNA to Develop Customized Therapies

AI's integration with **genomics** is one of the most exciting advancements in personalized medicine. **Genomics** is the study of genes, and through **genomic sequencing**, we can decode an individual's DNA to understand how their genetic makeup influences their health. AI's ability to process and analyze vast amounts of genomic data allows for the creation of highly **customized therapies** that are based on the individual's DNA.

1. Genomic Data Analysis

Human DNA contains approximately **3 billion base pairs**, and understanding the relationships between these genes and disease is a monumental task. Traditional methods of genetic research involved time-consuming manual analysis, which was limited in its ability to uncover hidden patterns within the data. But with AI, we can analyze genetic information on a much larger scale and with greater precision.

For example, in **oncology**, AI-powered genomic analysis can help doctors identify genetic mutations that are specific to a patient's type of cancer. In **breast cancer**, mutations in the **BRCA1** and **BRCA2** genes are associated with an increased risk of developing the disease. AI can analyze a patient's genomic data to identify these mutations, guiding the doctor to a more personalized treatment approach, such as a **preventative mastectomy** or **targeted chemotherapy**.

2. AI-Powered Drug Development for Genomic Mutations

One of the most powerful ways AI is being used in genomics is by helping to develop **customized therapies** based on genetic mutations. Let's take the example of **cystic fibrosis**, a genetic disorder that causes severe lung infections. In the past, treatments for cystic fibrosis were general and often ineffective. But AI is now being used to analyze the genetic mutations that cause cystic fibrosis, leading to the development of **targeted therapies** that focus on the specific mutation affecting the patient.

AI is not just helping to create targeted therapies—it's also enabling the development of **gene-editing technologies**, such as **CRISPR-Cas9**, which can directly alter an individual's DNA to correct genetic mutations. These advancements in genomics are making personalized treatments a reality for more and more patients every day.

Real-World Applications: AI-Guided Treatment Plans in Oncology, Cardiology, and Rare Diseases

Let's now explore some **real-world applications** of AI in personalized medicine, focusing on three key areas: **oncology, cardiology**, and **rare diseases**. In each of these fields, AI is playing a transformative role in how treatments are personalized and delivered.

1. Oncology: Personalized Cancer Treatment

Cancer treatment has long been a one-size-fits-all approach, but AI is now changing that. In **oncology**, AI is being used to develop **personalized treatment plans** by analyzing a patient's genetic data, lifestyle, and even environmental exposures. By looking at a patient's unique genetic mutations, AI can suggest treatments that are more likely to be effective.

For example, AI can analyze a breast cancer patient's **genetic mutations** and suggest targeted therapies, such as **HER2 inhibitors,** based on the patient's unique tumor profile. This level of personalization not only improves the likelihood of success but also minimizes the side effects that come with traditional chemotherapy.

2. Cardiology: Personalized Heart Disease Treatment

AI is also transforming **cardiology**, where it helps personalize treatments for patients with **heart disease**. AI systems analyze **genetic data**, **heart imaging**, and **lifestyle factors** to create treatment plans that are tailored to the individual's specific heart health. In **atrial fibrillation**, for example, AI analyzes a patient's genetic risk, lifestyle factors, and heart rhythm patterns to recommend the most effective treatment plan.

3. Rare Diseases: AI in Diagnosing and Treating Rare Conditions

AI is also proving to be a game-changer for patients with **rare diseases**. These conditions often go undiagnosed or misdiagnosed because they are so uncommon and symptoms can vary widely. AI algorithms, however, can analyze **genetic data** and **medical history** to identify patterns that may point to a rare disease, enabling doctors to make more accurate diagnoses.

For example, AI is being used to help identify rare **genetic disorders** like **Huntington's disease** or **Marfan syndrome**, which have similar symptoms but require different treatments. By analyzing a patient's DNA and comparing it with a vast database of known genetic disorders, AI can suggest the correct diagnosis and treatment plan.

Conclusion

The future of medicine lies in **personalization**—treatments designed just for you. **AI** is at the forefront of this revolution, enabling healthcare providers to offer treatments that are based not just on the disease but on your unique **genetic makeup**, **lifestyle**, and **environmental factors**. With the help of **AI and genomics**, we are now able to decode DNA and develop **customized therapies** that were once unimaginable. From **oncology** to **cardiology** and even rare diseases, AI is transforming the way we approach healthcare, making treatments more effective, safer, and tailored to the individual.

Personalized medicine is no longer a distant dream—it's here today, and with **AI**, it's becoming more accessible, more accurate, and more life-changing than ever before.

Chapter 6: AI in Surgery and Robotics

The Dawn of a New Era in Surgery

As I embarked on my travels across the globe, witnessing the remarkable strides being made in healthcare, one area that particularly stood out to me was the revolution taking place in **surgical medicine**. For centuries, surgery has been a delicate, highly skilled craft. Surgeons have relied on their hands, their intuition, and their years of practice to perform life-saving procedures. But today, thanks to the tremendous advancements in **Artificial Intelligence (AI)**, surgery is entering a new era—one where precision, speed, and minimally invasive techniques are transforming how surgeries are performed.

I recall visiting a leading hospital in **Switzerland**, known for its cutting-edge surgical techniques. There, I saw firsthand how **AI-powered robotic surgery** was being used to perform **complex procedures** with far greater accuracy than ever before. The surgeries were not only more precise but also less invasive, offering patients quicker recovery times and fewer complications.

As I stood there observing these highly advanced technologies in action, it became clear to me that AI in surgery is not just about enhancing the capabilities of **robotic systems**. It's about **empowering human surgeons** with tools that amplify their precision and intuition, making **surgery safer, more efficient, and more effective** than ever before.

In this chapter, I will take you through the incredible journey of how **AI** is transforming surgery—from robotic surgeries to the future of **autonomous procedures**. Together, we will explore the groundbreaking technologies that are reshaping the field and the potential they hold for revolutionizing healthcare.

AI-Powered Robotic Surgeries: Precision, Minimally Invasive, and Faster Recovery Times

The field of **robotic surgery** is one of the most tangible examples of AI's impact on the medical world. While **robotic surgeries** have been in existence for some time now, **AI** is rapidly accelerating their development, enhancing both their capabilities and accessibility. The fundamental promise of AI-powered robotic systems is to offer **increased precision, minimal invasiveness**, and **quicker recovery times** for patients.

How AI Robotics Work in Surgery

AI-powered robotic systems are equipped with sophisticated algorithms that allow them to learn from data and improve over time. These systems can integrate data from medical imaging, patient history, and real-time feedback from sensors to make precise adjustments during surgery. They can also **map out the surgical site** in 3D, helping surgeons visualize structures within the body with unprecedented clarity.

One of the most well-known robotic systems used today is the **da Vinci Surgical System**, which uses AI to assist surgeons in performing complex surgeries. These surgeries are typically done through **minimally invasive procedures**, meaning the surgeon can make small incisions instead of larger ones, which in turn leads to **faster recovery times** and **less pain** for the patient. The system also allows surgeons to operate with greater **precision**, reducing the chances of human error.

Real-World Example: Robotic Surgery for Prostate Cancer

I had the privilege of witnessing a **robotic prostatectomy** performed on a patient with prostate cancer in a **leading medical facility in the U.S.**. The procedure, traditionally a highly complex and delicate one, was performed using the **da Vinci robot** with AI assistance. The AI-powered system mapped the patient's anatomy, provided real-time feedback, and helped the surgeon navigate delicate tissues with remarkable accuracy.

Thanks to the robotic system's **precise movements** and **fine motor skills**, the surgeon was able to remove the tumor with minimal damage to surrounding tissue, which is often a challenge with traditional surgery. The patient was able to return home the next day and experienced significantly less pain compared to conventional open surgery, demonstrating the power of **AI-driven precision** in surgery.

Enhancing Surgeons' Capabilities with Augmented Reality and AI

Another key aspect of AI in surgery is its ability to **enhance the capabilities of human surgeons**. While robotic systems are incredibly powerful, the true magic happens when AI combines with **augmented reality (AR)** to provide surgeons with a **layer of visualization** that was once unthinkable.

AI and Augmented Reality: A Surgeon's New Eyes

With the help of AI-powered **augmented reality**, surgeons can now **visualize a patient's anatomy** in 3D, almost like a **virtual model**, overlaid onto the patient's body in real-time. AR systems use AI algorithms to analyze **medical imaging data**, such as **CT scans**, **MRIs**, and **X-rays**, and display these images directly in the surgeon's field of vision. This enables surgeons to see precisely where to cut, where the blood vessels are located, and how to approach the surgery with greater confidence.

For example, during a **spinal surgery**, AI can help the surgeon visualize the **spinal cord, bones,** and **nerves** in 3D. Using this real-time data, the surgeon can identify the exact position of the vertebrae and avoid damaging critical nerve structures, significantly reducing the risk of complications.

Real-World Example: Augmented Reality in Neurosurgery

One of the most fascinating examples I encountered was in a **neurosurgical procedure** in a hospital in **Germany**. The surgeon, equipped with an **AR headset,** could see a 3D model of the patient's brain overlaid onto their actual anatomy. As the surgery progressed, the AR system constantly updated the 3D model in real-time, providing the surgeon with a comprehensive view of the surgical site, including the location of blood vessels and critical brain areas.

This type of technology not only boosts the surgeon's confidence and efficiency but also helps improve patient outcomes by reducing the risk of human error. With AI-enhanced AR, **surgeons are able to make better decisions in real-time**, leading to safer and more effective surgeries.

The Future of Autonomous Surgeries: Opportunities and Challenges

As AI continues to evolve, many are asking: **Can we imagine a future where surgeries are entirely autonomous?** While this concept may seem futuristic, it is not as far-fetched as it once seemed. In fact, we are already seeing the early stages of

autonomous surgery in which AI systems operate with minimal or no human intervention.

The Promise of Autonomous Surgeries

Autonomous surgery refers to surgeries where **AI-powered robots** carry out the procedure with limited or no human oversight. These systems are designed to perform tasks such as **suturing, tissue removal**, and **incision making** based on pre-programmed protocols and real-time data analysis. Autonomous surgical robots are particularly suited for routine or repetitive procedures, which could reduce the risk of human fatigue and improve overall efficiency.

While there is still much to be done before fully autonomous surgeries become common, the potential benefits are undeniable. AI robots can work tirelessly, without the need for rest, and they can analyze vast amounts of data in real-time, making decisions based on the best available evidence.

Real-World Example: Autonomous Robotic Surgery in a Controlled Setting

In a **pioneering hospital** in the **U.K.**, an AI-powered robot was used to perform an initial test run of a **gallbladder removal surgery**. The robot was pre-programmed with a set of surgical guidelines, and it executed the procedure with minimal human oversight. Though a surgeon remained in the operating room to oversee the process, the robot performed the majority of the procedure autonomously, demonstrating the potential for **AI to handle routine tasks** efficiently.

While this technology is still in its infancy, it opens up exciting possibilities, especially in **remote areas** where skilled surgeons may not always be available. Autonomous robots could be deployed to **perform basic surgeries** in places where human resources are limited, improving access to life-saving healthcare.

Challenges of Autonomous Surgeries

However, the move toward fully autonomous surgeries raises important ethical and safety concerns. For instance, what happens if an AI system malfunctions during a critical procedure? How will liability be determined if a robot makes a mistake? And most importantly, how do we ensure that AI systems maintain the **human touch** that is so vital in healthcare?

Though the potential of autonomous surgeries is immense, these challenges must be carefully addressed before we can fully embrace this technology. For now, the focus remains on enhancing the surgeon's abilities with AI as an assistive tool, rather than replacing them entirely.

Other Areas of AI Integration in Surgery

Beyond robotic surgery, AI is making its mark in several other areas of surgical practice.

1. AI in Surgical Planning and Simulation

AI is also playing a vital role in **surgical planning**. Using data from **medical imaging**, AI systems can simulate different surgical approaches, allowing surgeons to choose the optimal method before stepping into the operating room. This kind of **pre-surgical simulation** is particularly useful in complex surgeries like **cardiac surgery** or **organ transplants**, where precision and planning are crucial.

2. AI in Post-Surgical Care

AI is also enhancing **post-surgical care**. After surgery, patients need constant monitoring to ensure they are recovering well. AI systems are increasingly being used to track patient recovery through **wearables** and **remote monitoring systems**. These systems can detect any signs of complications, such as infections or organ rejection, and alert medical staff before the problem becomes critical.

Conclusion: A Brave New World for Surgery

As we stand on the cusp of this transformative era in surgical medicine, it is clear that **AI is not replacing surgeons**; it is empowering them. With the help of AI-powered robotic systems, **augmented reality**, and the potential of autonomous surgery, surgeons are gaining **unprecedented levels of precision, efficiency, and safety** in the operating room.

While there are still hurdles to overcome, especially in fully autonomous surgeries, the future of surgery is incredibly promising. As AI continues to evolve, we will undoubtedly see more revolutionary advancements that will make surgeries faster, safer, and more effective—**ultimately benefiting patients around the world**.

For anyone involved in healthcare or the medical field, it's an exciting time to witness these advancements, and I'm thrilled to see how AI will continue to **reshape the landscape of surgery** in the years to come.

Chapter 7: AI in Preventive Healthcare and Wellness

Healthcare has always been about finding ways to cure and treat diseases, but what if we could shift the focus to **prevention**? What if, instead of waiting until a disease has progressed, we could **predict** it before it even begins? This is the future of healthcare, and it's unfolding right before our eyes thanks to the advancements in **Artificial Intelligence (AI)**.

During my travels and experiences across the globe, I've had the privilege of seeing the **transformation** that AI is bringing to the world of healthcare—not just in hospitals and clinics, but in **wellness and preventive care**. In every country I visited, one common thread emerged: there's a growing shift toward **wellness**, a movement away from reactive healthcare (treating diseases) and toward a more **proactive** approach (preventing diseases from occurring in the first place).

As someone who's deeply invested in AI and its potential to reshape industries, I'm excited to delve into one of the most **empowering aspects** of AI in healthcare: **preventive healthcare and wellness**. Through this chapter, I'll share how AI is **revolutionizing** our ability to predict, monitor, and improve health—long before a condition manifests itself.

From **predictive analytics** for early disease detection to **wearable devices** that monitor our health in real time, AI is helping us take control of our health in ways that were previously unimaginable. Let's explore how AI is not only **predicting health outcomes** but also **personalizing wellness** in a manner that is tailored specifically to each individual.

Copyright @2024 Jayant Deshmukh

Predictive Analytics for Early Detection of Diseases

One of the most exciting aspects of AI in **preventive healthcare** is its ability to use **predictive analytics** to **forecast potential health risks**. This is a game-changer, as it allows healthcare providers and individuals to detect diseases long before they exhibit symptoms, and in many cases, before they have even begun to take root.

How Predictive Analytics Works in Healthcare

At the heart of **predictive analytics** is the ability to analyze vast amounts of data—medical records, lifestyle factors, genetic information, and environmental influences—and identify patterns that signal potential health risks. AI algorithms can process this data much faster than the human brain, spotting trends and correlations that may not be immediately obvious to doctors.

Consider this: A **patient's medical history**, combined with **lifestyle factors** such as diet, exercise habits, and stress levels, can provide valuable insights into their likelihood of developing conditions like **diabetes**, **heart disease**, or even **cancer**. AI-driven predictive models can use this information to create a **risk profile**, allowing healthcare providers to take preemptive actions.

Real-World Example: AI in Predicting Heart Disease

A great example of **AI predictive analytics** comes from a **research study** I encountered in **Singapore**, where AI was used to predict the likelihood of a person developing **heart disease**. The study utilized a combination of **genetic data**, **lifestyle information**, and **medical imaging** to build a predictive model that could identify early signs of heart disease, even in patients with no obvious symptoms.

For instance, a person with high cholesterol levels, a sedentary lifestyle, and a family history of heart disease might show a **higher risk score** on an AI-powered predictive tool. The system then provides **personalized recommendations** for lifestyle changes—such as diet modification, exercise plans, or medications—that could significantly lower the individual's risk of developing heart disease.

What was truly inspiring about this technology was its **ability to empower individuals** to take control of their health. Instead of waiting for a crisis to happen, people could take **preventive actions** based on data-driven insights. AI has the potential to make us all more proactive about our health, rather than reactive.

Wearable Devices and Smart Sensors: Monitoring Health in Real-Time

Another monumental shift in healthcare is the rise of **wearable devices** and **smart sensors** that monitor our health in real time. Think of the fitness trackers we've seen so often—devices like **Fitbit**, **Apple Watch**, and **Oura Ring**—which have become common tools for tracking our steps, heart rate, sleep, and more. But these devices are now being powered by AI in ways that go beyond mere activity tracking.

How Wearable Devices Are Changing Healthcare

Today's **wearables** are not just simple pedometers. They're sophisticated health monitors that **continuously track a wide range of health metrics**, including heart rate, blood oxygen levels, body temperature, blood pressure, and even **blood sugar levels**. These devices collect vast amounts of data, and AI is at the heart of making sense of this information.

For example, AI algorithms in wearables can monitor a person's **heart rate variability** and detect irregularities that may indicate an underlying **cardiac issue**, such as **arrhythmia**. Similarly, AI can track fluctuations in a person's **blood pressure** and flag potential signs of **hypertension**—even if the person feels fine at the moment. Early detection of these issues can help patients seek timely medical attention, potentially preventing more severe health complications down the road.

Real-World Example: AI in Managing Chronic Conditions

In my travels, I came across a remarkable case in **California**, where AI-powered wearable devices were being used to help patients manage **chronic conditions** like **diabetes**. The device continuously monitored the patient's **blood glucose levels**, providing real-time feedback and suggestions for dietary changes or insulin adjustments.

What was fascinating about this system was that it wasn't just about data collection—it was about **actionable insights**. The AI wasn't simply logging the data but **analyzing trends** and **predicting future changes**. For example, it could alert the patient that their glucose levels were trending toward a dangerous range before they even noticed any symptoms, giving them time to take corrective action.

This kind of **real-time health monitoring** provides **valuable insights** that can help individuals stay on top of their health and prevent complications before they occur. Moreover, it allows for more **personalized care**, with healthcare providers able to offer tailored recommendations based on the data collected by wearables.

AI-Enabled Lifestyle Management: Personalized Fitness and Nutrition Programs

As AI continues to evolve, it's also changing the way we think about **wellness**. The concept of wellness isn't just about being free from disease; it's about achieving a state of **optimal health**, and AI is helping individuals tailor their wellness journey through **personalized fitness and nutrition programs**.

AI and Fitness: Personalized Exercise Plans

We all know that **exercise** is crucial for maintaining good health, but it's often difficult to know where to start or how to tailor a fitness plan to our individual needs. This is where AI comes in. Through the use of **AI-powered fitness apps** and devices, individuals can now receive **personalized workout routines** based on their **fitness levels**, **goals**, and even **genetic predispositions**.

I had the opportunity to observe a **fitness startup in London** that was using AI to create **customized fitness programs**. The AI system analyzed the user's **current fitness data**, such as their strength, flexibility, and endurance, and then generated a personalized workout plan that was optimized for **maximum results**. Over time, the AI adjusted the plan based on the user's progress, ensuring that the program evolved as they got fitter.

What was truly revolutionary about this was that it wasn't just a one-size-fits-all approach. The AI was capable of **adapting** to each person's unique body and needs, making exercise more accessible and effective for people of all fitness levels.

AI and Nutrition: Tailored Meal Plans

Nutrition plays an equally important role in our overall wellness. Yet, with so many conflicting dietary trends and misinformation, it can be overwhelming to know what to eat. AI is helping to take the guesswork out of nutrition by offering **personalized meal plans** based on a person's **genetic makeup, lifestyle,** and **health goals**.

Take, for example, a **nutrition app** I came across in **New York**, where AI analyzed users' **blood sugar levels, weight,** and **activity levels** to create a **tailored meal plan**. The app even suggested recipes that were nutritionally balanced and aligned with the user's health goals, such as weight loss, muscle gain, or improving gut health.

By **integrating genetic data** (such as information on lactose intolerance, food sensitivities, or predispositions to certain conditions like high cholesterol), AI can provide even more **targeted** and **scientifically backed** recommendations for what to eat.

Other Areas of AI in Preventive Healthcare and Wellness

1. Mental Health and AI: Early Detection of Mental Health Disorders

AI is also making strides in **mental health**. Predictive models are now being used to detect signs of mental health conditions, such as **depression, anxiety,** and **bipolar disorder**, based on data from **social media activity, speech patterns,** and **psychological assessments**. AI algorithms can analyze these signals to predict the onset of mental health issues, allowing for early intervention and support.

2. AI in Environmental Health Monitoring

In some areas of the world, AI is being used to monitor **environmental factors** that can impact health, such as **air**

quality and **pollution levels.** By tracking air quality in real time, AI systems can predict the health risks associated with poor air quality and provide **personalized health advice** to people who may be at higher risk, such as those with respiratory conditions.

Conclusion: The Promise of AI in Preventive Healthcare and Wellness

The integration of AI in **preventive healthcare and wellness** represents one of the most exciting transformations in the healthcare sector today. By harnessing the power of **predictive analytics, wearables,** and **personalized health plans,** AI is empowering us to take control of our health like never before. Whether it's preventing diseases before they happen, optimizing our fitness and nutrition, or monitoring our health in real time, AI is helping us live healthier, longer lives.

As we continue to embrace AI in preventive healthcare, it's important to remember that we are not replacing the human touch—we are **augmenting** it. With AI, we have the potential to achieve **a future where healthcare is truly personalized**, where each person can receive the **right care at the right time** based on their unique needs and circumstances.

The road ahead is full of possibilities, and I am excited to see where AI will take us on this journey toward better health and wellness for all.

Chapter 8: AI in Patient Engagement and Experience

One of the most profound changes AI is bringing to healthcare is in **patient engagement**—the way patients interact with healthcare providers, how they manage their health, and how they experience care. The traditional healthcare system has often been seen as disjointed and impersonal, where patients feel like just another number in a long list of appointments. However, AI is revolutionizing this narrative, offering tools that bring **efficiency**, **personalization**, and **convenience** to the forefront of patient care.

Through my years of exploring global healthcare systems and witnessing firsthand how AI is transforming the industry, I've come to realize how technology, when applied thoughtfully, can significantly enhance a patient's experience. Imagine a world where you have **instant access** to medical advice, the ability to schedule an appointment at your convenience, and personalized reminders to ensure you never miss a medication dose. This world is already here, and it's being shaped by **AI-driven virtual assistants, chatbots,** and **personalized patient engagement tools**.

In this chapter, we will explore how AI is not just **transforming patient care** in the clinical sense but is also enhancing the **overall patient experience**. From providing real-time support through virtual health assistants to optimizing the journey with personalized reminders and feedback systems, AI is creating a more **engaged, empowered,** and **satisfied patient base**.

AI-Driven Virtual Health Assistants: 24/7 Support for Patients

In the past, accessing healthcare advice and information often required **appointments, long wait times**, and **inconvenient office hours**. But now, with the advent of **AI-driven virtual health assistants**, patients have the ability to receive immediate assistance, no matter where they are or what time it is.

The Rise of Virtual Health Assistants

AI-powered virtual assistants are changing the way patients interact with healthcare services. These digital assistants, powered by **Natural Language Processing (NLP)** and **Machine Learning (ML)**, can provide users with instant answers to their health queries, book appointments, track medication schedules, and offer guidance on managing chronic conditions.

I had the privilege of witnessing how a healthcare startup in **San Francisco** integrated an AI-driven virtual health assistant into their system. Their assistant was available to patients **24/7**, providing answers to general medical questions, offering advice on managing conditions like **hypertension** or **diabetes**, and reminding patients to take their medications. This assistant wasn't just a tool—it was a **constant companion** that provided personalized support, regardless of time or location.

The beauty of this AI assistant is that it uses the information from a patient's **health records** and **preferences** to tailor responses. For example, if a patient with diabetes inquires about what they should eat, the assistant can provide personalized dietary suggestions based on their specific condition and past conversations. Moreover, these assistants are **always available**, making healthcare more **accessible** than ever before.

Chatbots for Symptom Checking and Appointment Scheduling

While virtual health assistants provide continuous support, **AI-powered chatbots** are another area where technology is improving the patient experience. These intelligent bots can help patients navigate the often-overwhelming process of **symptom checking**, **diagnostic guidance**, and **appointment scheduling**.

Symptom Checking with AI

Many patients face challenges in determining whether their symptoms are serious enough to seek medical attention. In the past, this often meant **waiting days for an appointment** or visiting the **emergency room** for something that might have been treatable with simpler interventions. Enter AI-driven chatbots that help patients assess their symptoms in real-time and provide them with guidance on the next best steps.

For instance, I recall a healthcare initiative in **India**, where an AI-powered chatbot was deployed in underserved areas to help people identify early symptoms of common diseases, such as **flu**, **COVID-19**, or **gastrointestinal disorders**. The chatbot would prompt the user with a series of questions, asking about **fever**, **fatigue**, **cough**, or other symptoms, and then use the responses to suggest whether the patient should consult a healthcare professional or manage the symptoms at home.

This kind of symptom checking reduces unnecessary hospital visits and allows patients to make more informed decisions about their health, significantly improving their experience with the healthcare system.

Appointment Scheduling Made Easy

Gone are the days of long phone calls to schedule an appointment or waiting weeks for availability. **AI chatbots** can now offer patients a seamless and efficient way to schedule their appointments. By connecting to a **provider's calendar**, these bots allow patients to check available slots in real-time and book their visits instantly.

Take, for example, a hospital in **Germany** that integrated an AI chatbot into their patient portal. Instead of waiting on hold for an appointment, patients simply interacted with the bot to select their preferred date and time. The AI assistant also offered reminders, rescheduling options, and pre-appointment instructions, ensuring that the entire process was **hassle-free** and **user-friendly**. This streamlined approach not only saved time for patients but also improved the efficiency of the healthcare provider's administrative team.

Enhancing the Patient Journey: Personalized Reminders and Feedback Systems

The patient journey, from diagnosis to treatment, can be overwhelming, especially when it involves managing chronic conditions or undergoing long-term treatments. AI is now playing a crucial role in helping patients stay on top of their healthcare journey through **personalized reminders** and **feedback systems**.

Personalized Reminders: Never Miss a Dose or Appointment

Medication adherence is one of the greatest challenges in healthcare, particularly for patients with chronic conditions who need to take multiple medications at specific times. AI can help solve this problem by providing **personalized medication** reminders tailored to the patient's schedule. These reminders can be delivered via text messages, smartphone notifications, or even through voice assistants like Amazon's Alexa or Google Assistant.

I remember hearing about a patient in **New York** who was managing **rheumatoid arthritis**. With the help of a **smartphone app** powered by AI, the patient received automated reminders to take their medication, along with tips on managing their condition. The app also tracked medication adherence and sent reminders to **refill prescriptions** when necessary. These reminders not only helped the patient maintain consistency in their treatment but also made them feel **more in control** of their health.

Real-Time Feedback Systems

Another fascinating application of AI in patient engagement is its ability to offer **real-time feedback**. Whether it's tracking progress after surgery, monitoring vital signs during treatment, or providing insights on recovery after a health scare, AI-driven feedback systems are becoming a valuable tool in improving the patient experience.

For example, in a **hospital in Sweden**, patients undergoing **post-operative care** received real-time feedback through an AI-powered platform. The system would monitor their vital signs, provide feedback on **wound healing**, and offer suggestions for improving mobility. If the system detected any irregularities or signs of complications, it immediately notified healthcare providers, enabling them to intervene early and prevent further issues.

These real-time feedback systems are **reassuring** for patients and help them feel more **connected** to their healthcare team throughout their recovery.

AI and Emotional Support: A Personal Connection

Healthcare isn't just about physical symptoms—it's also about the **emotional journey** patients face. Navigating illness or managing a chronic condition can be emotionally taxing, and many patients often feel **isolated** or **anxious**. AI is helping to bridge this emotional gap by providing **emotional support** to patients in ways that are both empathetic and responsive.

AI as a Virtual Companion

In some regions, healthcare systems have introduced **AI companions** that help patients cope with the emotional challenges of illness. These virtual companions use conversational AI to engage with patients, offer words of encouragement, and even provide mindfulness exercises to reduce stress.

A **mental health app in the UK**, for example, uses AI to engage users in daily conversations about their mental health, offering advice on coping mechanisms and providing emotional support. If the user exhibits signs of severe anxiety or depression, the AI system can direct them to appropriate resources or emergency help, ensuring they don't feel alone during a difficult time.

The Future of AI in Patient Engagement and Experience

The potential for AI to transform patient engagement and experience is vast. As technology continues to evolve, we can expect even more **advanced solutions** to enhance every aspect of the patient journey, including:

- **AI-powered predictive models** that suggest the best course of treatment based on the patient's health history and genetic data.
- **Enhanced personalized care** using AI to adjust treatment plans in real-time based on patient responses.
- **Integration with wearable devices** for seamless tracking of health metrics and ongoing engagement with healthcare providers.

As we move forward, the focus will be on **creating a seamless, integrated experience** for patients—one where AI works in harmony with healthcare providers to ensure that patients not only receive the best possible care but also feel **heard, understood**, and **supported** throughout their entire healthcare journey.

Conclusion: A New Era of Patient Engagement

AI has the power to change not just the way we **diagnose** and **treat** diseases but also the way we **interact with** and **experience** healthcare. By integrating **virtual assistants, chatbots**, and **personalized feedback systems**, AI is giving patients more control, more information, and more **empowerment** over their own health.

As I have seen firsthand, the promise of AI in patient engagement is not just about technology—it's about **building a more compassionate, efficient, and accessible healthcare system**. One where patients feel that they are not only receiving care but are actively involved in their health decisions, supported by a system that is **always available** to guide them.

The future of healthcare is exciting, and as AI continues to evolve, the patient experience will become more **personalized, efficient,** and **supportive** than ever before. The journey has only just begun, and I am eager to see where it takes us.

Chapter 9: AI in Healthcare Administration and Operations

As we've delved into the many ways AI is transforming direct patient care, there's another aspect of healthcare that's equally important—**healthcare administration and operations**. This often-overlooked side of the industry is critical for ensuring that healthcare systems function efficiently and that resources are used optimally. AI is playing a huge role in **streamlining operations, optimizing resource management**, and **enhancing decision-making** at every level, from hospital management to supply chain logistics.

When we think of AI in healthcare, we usually envision smart diagnostic tools or robotic surgeries. However, AI's true power is also in the unseen layers of healthcare—those behind-the-scenes systems that ensure hospitals, clinics, and healthcare facilities run smoothly and are able to meet patient demand without unnecessary waste. This chapter will explore how AI is transforming **healthcare administration**, from optimizing **hospital management** to improving **supply chain management** and **predictive analytics**. We'll also look at how these technologies can make healthcare more affordable, sustainable, and accessible to everyone.

Streamlining Hospital Management: Optimizing Resources and Reducing Waste

Hospital management is a complex puzzle—one that requires coordinating between **doctors, nurses, administrative staff,** and countless **departments** to ensure that patients receive timely and effective care. But with the demands placed on modern healthcare systems, there is a constant need to optimize resources and reduce inefficiencies. AI can help healthcare facilities achieve this by offering **data-driven solutions** for smarter decision-making.

AI in Staff Scheduling and Resource Allocation

Let me tell you about a hospital I visited in **Tokyo**, Japan, where AI had been implemented to streamline its staff scheduling. Hospitals, especially larger ones, face the challenge of ensuring the right staff is available at the right time. Mismanagement of staff schedules can lead to **overworked staff, delayed treatments**, and a **reduced quality of care**. On the other hand, **understaffing** creates significant problems, especially during peak hours or public health crises.

The hospital in Tokyo integrated an AI-powered **staff scheduling system** that analyzed patient volume, staff availability, and historical data to optimize nurse and doctor shifts. The AI was able to predict busy periods based on previous trends and allocate more staff to critical areas, such as the emergency room or intensive care unit. This resulted in a **significant reduction in wait times, improved patient care**, and a more **balanced workload** for hospital staff. The system was also designed to adjust for unexpected changes, such as sudden surges in patient numbers, making the hospital **flexible** and **adaptive** to real-time needs.

Moreover, AI can assist in resource allocation. For instance, **machine learning algorithms** can track hospital inventories—such as medications, medical supplies, and equipment—and predict which items will be needed and when. This predictive analysis reduces **waste, overstocking**, and the risk of **running out of critical supplies** at the wrong time.

Predictive Analytics for Patient Flow and Demand Forecasting

Patient flow management is another critical aspect of healthcare administration that AI is changing. Hospitals are busy places, and managing the flow of patients through various stages of care is a complicated task. Efficient patient flow ensures that **patients receive timely care**, **beds are utilized optimally**, and **discharge processes** are smooth and hassle-free.

Optimizing Bed Management

One of the hospitals I visited in **London** utilized AI to manage patient flow through predictive analytics. By analyzing historical data, the AI system could predict how many patients would be admitted on any given day, based on trends and factors like **seasonal illnesses**, **regional outbreaks**, and **public health events**. This data allowed the hospital to **forecast demand** for resources such as ICU beds, general hospital beds, and surgical theaters.

If the system predicted an influx of patients in a particular department, administrators could quickly adjust staffing levels and prepare for the increased demand. In contrast, during off-peak periods, the system would suggest **discharge planning** to make the best use of available beds. This led to better **patient care**, as beds were always available for critical patients, and the hospital **avoided overcapacity** and **delays in care**.

The same predictive tools were used for **emergency departments (EDs)**, where AI models could predict when certain types of **medical emergencies** were more likely based on time of day, weather patterns, or even local events. Knowing this, hospitals could plan and allocate emergency staff more effectively, ultimately **improving patient outcomes** and **reducing overcrowding** in EDs.

Demand Forecasting and Scheduling

Moreover, AI is enhancing demand forecasting, not only in terms of patient volume but also the services patients will need. For example, AI can predict which types of treatments and procedures will be in demand at different times of the year. This allows **healthcare managers** to plan their budgets and procurement strategies accordingly. If an AI system predicts a higher demand for **orthopedic surgeries** due to winter-related injuries, the hospital can schedule the necessary equipment, surgical staff, and medical supplies in advance.

This foresight helps eliminate **bottlenecks**, ensuring that the healthcare system is always prepared to meet patient needs efficiently.

Enhancing Supply Chain Management: Ensuring Availability of Medicines and Equipment

Supply chain management is one area where inefficiencies can lead to critical shortages or overstocking of medical supplies and medications. Hospitals must maintain a delicate balance between **avoiding shortages** and **avoiding waste**. The role of AI in **healthcare supply chain management** is crucial to making this process more efficient, especially when it comes to **predicting** and **managing inventories**.

AI-Powered Inventory Management

One example of AI revolutionizing supply chain management is in a **hospital in the Netherlands**, where the integration of AI in inventory management drastically reduced waste while ensuring that medications and equipment were always available when needed. The hospital used AI-powered systems that continuously monitored and analyzed data from various departments to assess the **demand for supplies** in real-time.

For instance, if the system detected that a certain medication was being used in larger quantities for treating respiratory illnesses due to a sudden spike in flu cases, it would automatically alert the hospital's procurement team to order more of that medication. In this way, the AI system allowed the hospital to adjust supply orders based on real-time data and **demand fluctuations**, ensuring a **steady supply** of necessary resources without overstocking or facing shortages.

In addition to managing pharmaceutical supplies, AI is being used to ensure that critical medical equipment, such as **ventilators**, **defibrillators**, and **surgical instruments**, is available and functioning. AI systems can predict when equipment is likely to need maintenance or when it's nearing the end of its useful life, enabling healthcare organizations to perform timely repairs or replacements before any **downtime** occurs.

AI for Financial Management: Reducing Costs and Improving Efficiency

Healthcare organizations are often burdened with rising operational costs and the need for sustainable financial practices. AI's role in **financial management** within healthcare can reduce costs, improve budget forecasting, and streamline administrative processes.

Cost Optimization Through AI

In a **hospital in Singapore**, AI was employed to monitor and optimize spending across various departments, including patient care, operations, and administrative functions. The system analyzed patterns of spending, identified areas of waste, and suggested more cost-efficient solutions. For example, AI could help hospitals identify areas where energy consumption was unnecessarily high, leading to actionable insights on how to reduce energy costs without compromising patient care.

Furthermore, AI is aiding in **fraud detection** and **billing errors**, which are common challenges in healthcare. AI systems can automatically analyze billing data to flag any inconsistencies, ensuring that insurance claims are processed more efficiently and accurately, thus reducing the risk of **financial loss**.

Improving Patient and Staff Satisfaction Through AI

AI is also playing a role in enhancing **staff and patient satisfaction** by eliminating administrative burdens. In many healthcare organizations, administrative tasks such as **data entry**, **scheduling**, and **documentation** take up a significant portion of both **doctor's** and **nurse's** time. By using **AI tools** to automate routine tasks, healthcare providers can free up valuable time for patient care, leading to **better job satisfaction** and **higher-quality care**.

For example, **voice recognition software** powered by AI is now being used to assist doctors with dictating patient notes, allowing them to spend more time with patients instead of typing. This technology not only improves **efficiency** but also **reduces burnout** among healthcare workers.

Copyright @2024 Jayant Deshmukh

The Future of AI in Healthcare Administration

The potential for AI to optimize healthcare administration is enormous. As technology advances, we can expect even more **integrated systems** that bring together patient data, staff schedules, supply chains, and financial management into **unified platforms**. These platforms will be powered by advanced machine learning algorithms, capable of **anticipating needs, forecasting demands,** and **providing real-time solutions**.

Moreover, as healthcare systems around the world continue to adopt AI, we will see more **interoperability** between AI solutions in different institutions, allowing for **cross-hospital collaborations** and **better resource distribution** across regions.

Conclusion: Shaping a More Efficient and Sustainable Healthcare System

AI's impact on healthcare administration and operations is not just about **increasing efficiency**—it's about creating a more **affordable, sustainable,** and **accessible** healthcare system. By optimizing hospital management, predicting patient flow, and improving supply chain logistics, AI helps healthcare providers offer better care at lower costs, while **reducing waste** and **improving patient outcomes**.

As we look ahead, it's clear that AI will continue to play a pivotal role in shaping the future of healthcare. It's not just about making hospitals run more smoothly; it's about **improving the overall patient experience**, enhancing the **workplace environment** for healthcare professionals, and ultimately creating a system that is more **effective** and **inclusive** for everyone.

The AI-driven revolution in healthcare administration and operations is well underway, and it's an exciting time to witness these changes that will benefit **patients, providers,** and **healthcare organizations** alike.

Chapter 10: AI in Global Health and Public Health Challenges

A Global Perspective on AI in Health

Throughout the world, healthcare systems are facing immense pressure from a variety of challenges, both new and persistent. From rising costs to infectious disease outbreaks, there is an urgent need for solutions that can **bridge the gap** between **healthcare access** and **quality of care**. In the past, many public health challenges seemed insurmountable. But in the age of Artificial Intelligence (AI), we now have a unique opportunity to address these issues in ways that were previously unimaginable.

AI, with its ability to **process vast amounts of data**, **predict future trends**, and **optimize healthcare resources**, is now at the forefront of solving some of the world's most pressing health challenges. In this chapter, we will explore how AI is being used to tackle global health crises, improve access to healthcare in underserved regions, and address health inequities worldwide.

AI's Role in Tackling Pandemics: Predicting Outbreaks and Managing Resources

The COVID-19 Pandemic: A Wake-Up Call

The world's response to the **COVID-19 pandemic** demonstrated just how unprepared we were for a global health crisis. Hospitals were overwhelmed, resources were stretched thin, and millions of lives were lost. But in the midst of this unprecedented challenge, AI emerged as a powerful tool in helping to **predict outbreaks**, **track the virus**, and **manage healthcare resources**.

I remember hearing from colleagues in **Italy**, one of the hardest-hit countries during the early stages of the pandemic. The healthcare system was on the brink of collapse. Yet, at the same time, AI-driven platforms were working behind the scenes to **analyze real-time data** on infection rates, predict where the virus would spread next, and optimize the allocation of resources like **ventilators, medical staff, and ICU beds**.

AI-Driven Predictive Models: A New Era in Pandemic Preparedness

AI-powered **predictive models** proved crucial in the fight against COVID-19. These models, which used machine learning algorithms, **analyzed patterns of disease spread** and helped authorities predict future outbreaks. For instance, AI systems that analyzed travel data, population density, and historical disease trends were able to identify high-risk areas and predict where new outbreaks were likely to occur. This allowed governments and health organizations to **deploy resources** and **preventive measures** more effectively.

In **Singapore**, a machine learning model helped identify emerging outbreaks weeks before they were officially detected. The model combined real-time surveillance data with environmental and demographic factors to predict where new COVID-19 clusters would arise. By analyzing the movement of people and the spread of infections in real time, AI gave governments the foresight needed to **manage health resources** efficiently, limit the spread of the virus, and **impose targeted lockdowns**.

These AI-driven systems also played a role in identifying new mutations of the virus. AI algorithms could **analyze genetic sequences** of viral samples and track mutations, allowing for quicker detection of more infectious variants. This was essential for **vaccine development, treatment protocols**, and **public health responses**.

Improving Access to Healthcare in Underserved Regions through AI-Powered Telemedicine

Telemedicine: Bridging the Gap

One of the most significant advancements during the pandemic was the rapid growth of **telemedicine**—a service that uses AI-powered tools and platforms to connect patients with healthcare providers remotely. The pandemic underscored the need for telemedicine, especially in **underserved regions** where access to healthcare facilities is limited.

In **rural India**, where healthcare access can be scarce, telemedicine platforms powered by AI have made a tremendous impact. I saw this firsthand during my travels to villages in the Indian subcontinent. Here, AI-enabled systems are used to provide **remote consultations**, allowing doctors to diagnose and treat patients from hundreds of miles away. For example, in some regions, **AI-based chatbots** ask patients a series of questions about their symptoms, analyze the responses, and suggest potential diagnoses. This is followed by a **video consultation** with a doctor, who then confirms the diagnosis and provides treatment options.

AI-driven telemedicine is particularly beneficial in regions with limited medical infrastructure. In **Kenya**, for instance, a telemedicine system equipped with AI tools helps healthcare providers conduct remote consultations, monitor patient health, and even deliver **mental health support**. AI platforms assess patients' symptoms and determine whether they need immediate attention or can manage with self-care. This not only improves access to healthcare but also reduces the burden on local clinics and hospitals.

In **remote areas of Sub-Saharan Africa**, where healthcare workers are scarce, AI systems are helping to fill this gap by offering **virtual healthcare support**. AI platforms analyze patient data from wearable devices, provide predictive alerts about potential health issues, and guide patients on when to seek in-person medical care. This **remote monitoring** can drastically reduce mortality rates from conditions like **diabetes**, **hypertension**, and **malaria**, which are prevalent in these regions.

Addressing Health Inequities: AI's Potential to Bridge the Gap

The Challenge of Health Inequities

One of the most profound challenges facing healthcare today is the **disparity in healthcare access**. Whether it's due to geography, socioeconomic status, or other factors, millions of people around the world are denied the quality healthcare they deserve. This is especially true in **low-income** and **developing nations**, where inadequate healthcare infrastructure and **limited resources** lead to health outcomes that are far worse than in wealthier countries.

I've witnessed this inequality during my travels to **South America** and **Africa**, where communities with limited access to healthcare facilities often suffer from preventable diseases. **AI has the potential** to **bridge this gap** and ensure that everyone, regardless of their location or socioeconomic status, can access high-quality care.

AI for Health Equity: Breaking Down Barriers

AI's role in improving healthcare equity is multifaceted, but perhaps one of its most significant contributions is **resource optimization**. By leveraging AI, **low-resource healthcare systems** can function more efficiently and effectively. For example, in **rural Africa**, where access to healthcare professionals is limited, AI-powered diagnostic tools can enable **remote consultations** with doctors, allowing patients to get diagnoses and treatment plans without having to travel long distances.

In **Brazil**, a country with vast disparities in healthcare access, AI is being used to **reduce wait times** for critical procedures in underserved regions. Machine learning models analyze patient histories, **predict healthcare demands**, and automatically schedule patients based on the urgency of their medical needs. This has **improved efficiency**, ensured that **no patient is left behind**, and reduced the burden on healthcare providers.

Furthermore, AI tools that detect **health risks**, such as **early-stage cancers** or **heart conditions**, can help identify at-risk individuals in **disadvantaged communities**. Early detection in **rural** and **low-income urban areas** can save lives that might otherwise be lost due to delayed diagnosis.

AI for Targeted Health Interventions

In **Bangladesh**, a program called **AI for Health Equity** used AI algorithms to identify **underprivileged populations** that were most at risk for diseases like **tuberculosis**. The AI analyzed **data from health surveys**, **hospital records**, and **public health data** to pinpoint where interventions were most needed. Based on these findings, healthcare workers were deployed to provide **early** screening, vaccinations, and treatments, significantly reducing the disease's impact in these communities.

The technology is also being used to improve **maternal health** in underserved regions. **AI-driven systems** can assess data from pregnant women, such as their **medical history, age**, and **pre-existing conditions**, to predict complications that might arise during childbirth. This allows healthcare workers to take **preventive measures** and ensure that **pregnant women** in rural or impoverished areas receive the **care they need** before it's too late.

AI in Global Health Initiatives: Shaping the Future of Healthcare Access

AI is transforming the way global health initiatives are planned, funded, and executed. Through international collaborations, AI is helping to **optimize resource distribution** and **prioritize interventions** in areas where they are needed the most. AI tools enable organizations such as the **World Health Organization (WHO)** and **Doctors Without Borders** to track health trends across the globe, predict disease outbreaks, and allocate resources accordingly.

Moreover, AI can make health interventions more **cost-effective**. By automating administrative tasks, reducing waste, and increasing the accuracy of diagnoses, AI can reduce the financial burden on global health organizations and ensure that more resources are channeled directly into patient care.

Conclusion: A Future of Equity and Access for All

AI holds tremendous promise in addressing the world's most significant public health challenges. From **predicting pandemics** to **improving healthcare access** in underserved regions, AI is transforming how we approach global health. While much remains to be done, the potential for AI to **bridge healthcare gaps** and **ensure equitable access** to quality care is limitless. As we continue to develop and integrate AI into healthcare systems worldwide, it's clear that the future of global health is brighter, more accessible, and more inclusive than ever before.

Through AI, we have the chance to build a healthcare system that not only responds to crises but also actively **improves health outcomes**, **addresses inequities**, and **ensures universal access** to the care we all deserve. The next chapter in global health is already being written, and AI is leading the way.

Chapter 11: Ethical and Regulatory Challenges in AI-Driven Healthcare

Navigating the Path of Innovation and Ethics

As Artificial Intelligence (AI) continues to revolutionize healthcare, one thing becomes increasingly clear: with great power comes great responsibility. The rapid integration of AI into healthcare systems brings tremendous promise, from improving diagnostic accuracy to optimizing patient care and predicting disease outbreaks. However, alongside these breakthroughs lie significant **ethical and regulatory challenges** that must be addressed to ensure the responsible and equitable use of AI in healthcare.

I remember, during my travels to various healthcare hubs across the world, discussing with doctors, AI engineers, and policymakers about the exciting opportunities AI brings to the medical field. But one recurring concern among them was **how to balance the pursuit of innovation with ethical considerations**. Many expressed the need to safeguard **patient rights**, **privacy**, and **equity**, ensuring that AI systems serve **all people** fairly and transparently.

In this chapter, we'll explore the ethical issues surrounding AI in healthcare, the **regulatory frameworks** governing its use, and how the industry can address these challenges to maximize AI's potential while protecting public trust.

Balancing Innovation with Ethical Considerations: Data Privacy, Security, and Biases

Data Privacy and Security: The Cornerstone of Trust

One of the most fundamental ethical considerations when integrating AI into healthcare is **data privacy**. Healthcare systems are powered by **vast amounts of sensitive data**—from patient histories and diagnoses to genetic information and treatment plans. The power of AI comes from its ability to analyze these large datasets to uncover insights that can improve care. But when it comes to personal health information, the question arises: How can we ensure that this data is secure and used responsibly?

During my conversations with healthcare professionals in the **United States**, many emphasized the challenge of protecting patient data amidst increasing cyber threats. **Data breaches** in healthcare are unfortunately common, with hackers targeting healthcare organizations for valuable personal information. This is why **data encryption** and **strong security protocols** must be integrated into AI systems from the ground up. I recall one particular instance when a health organization had to deal with the fallout of a data breach. The trust that patients had in the system was severely compromised, and AI systems that could have improved care became secondary to the task of rebuilding that trust.

AI systems must adhere to strict **data protection laws** like the **General Data Protection Regulation (GDPR)** in the European Union or the **Health Insurance Portability and Accountability Act (HIPAA)** in the United States. These laws are designed to **protect patient privacy**, limit access to personal data, and ensure that any data used by AI algorithms is anonymized, encrypted, and properly safeguarded. For AI to succeed in healthcare, patient trust must be earned, and that begins with **data security**.

The Challenge of Bias in AI Systems

Another pressing ethical concern in AI-driven healthcare is the potential for **bias** in algorithms. **Biases** can arise at any stage of the AI development process, from the selection of training data to the design of the algorithm itself. If AI systems are trained on biased datasets, they can perpetuate and even amplify existing inequalities in healthcare.

Let me share an example from my travels in **India**. During a visit to a hospital in a rural area, I observed the incredible potential of AI systems to help doctors diagnose diseases like tuberculosis and malaria. However, one healthcare worker pointed out an issue: the **AI model** was primarily trained using data from urban populations, leading to a system that didn't perform as well for rural patients. The **algorithm** failed to account for certain environmental and lifestyle factors unique to rural areas, leading to a **lower accuracy** in diagnostics. This revealed a critical flaw: the data used to train AI systems must be **diverse, inclusive**, and representative of the populations that the technology serves.

Bias in AI can also emerge in areas like **treatment recommendations**. For example, if an AI algorithm is trained on data that primarily includes treatments for one gender, race, or age group, it may not provide accurate or equitable recommendations for other groups. In **healthcare, this can** have serious consequences—leading to misdiagnoses, ineffective treatments, and even harm to patients.

Addressing Bias in AI: A Step-by-Step Approach

1. **Diverse Data Sets**: The first step in addressing bias is to ensure that the data used to train AI systems is **diverse** and **representative** of all patient demographics. This includes considering **race**, **age**, **gender**, **socioeconomic status**, and **geographic location**. By including a broad range of data, we can mitigate the risk of bias and

improve the AI's ability to make fair and accurate recommendations for everyone.

2. **Bias Detection Tools**: AI developers need to integrate **bias detection tools** into the development process. These tools can help identify and mitigate biases in datasets and algorithms before they are deployed in healthcare settings.

3. **Continuous Monitoring**: Once deployed, AI systems should be **constantly monitored** for performance discrepancies across different patient groups. If certain groups are being underserved or misdiagnosed, adjustments must be made to the algorithm.

4. **Transparency and Accountability**: AI companies must be transparent about how their algorithms work, the data they are trained on, and the steps they are taking to reduce bias. This transparency will help build trust and ensure that AI systems are used responsibly.

The Importance of Explainable AI in Healthcare Decision-Making

What is Explainable AI?

As AI becomes more integral to healthcare, another ethical concern emerges: **explainability**. When AI makes decisions about patient care—such as suggesting a treatment or predicting disease outcomes—it is critical that healthcare professionals and patients can **understand** how those decisions were made. This is where **explainable AI** (XAI) comes into play.

Explainable AI refers to AI systems that provide clear, understandable explanations for their decisions. In healthcare, this is especially important because doctors and patients must feel confident that the AI is making accurate and fair decisions. If an AI algorithm suggests a treatment plan for a patient, doctors need to know **why** the system came to that conclusion.

I had the privilege of discussing this topic with a **healthcare startup** in **Germany** that was developing AI solutions for personalized cancer treatment. They shared how they had integrated **explainability** into their AI system by ensuring that it could provide detailed, step-by-step explanations for every decision it made. For instance, if the AI recommended a specific chemotherapy regimen, the system would explain how it arrived at that decision, citing relevant patient data, medical literature, and statistical probabilities.

The Need for Explainability in Patient Care

Without explainability, AI systems risk becoming "black boxes" that even the healthcare professionals who use them cannot understand. This is particularly concerning in critical healthcare settings, where treatment decisions can have life-or-death consequences.

Doctors need to be able to trust and verify AI's decision-making process. They need to know if the AI's recommendation is based on **sound evidence**, and they need to be able to explain it to the patient. This is especially important in situations involving **complex treatments**, such as cancer therapies, where patients may have multiple options and need to make informed decisions.

International Regulatory Standards for AI Adoption in Healthcare

The Need for Regulation

AI in healthcare is still a relatively new field, and as such, it is not always subject to comprehensive regulatory oversight. However, given the potential risks and ethical concerns, there is a growing demand for clear, international **regulatory standards** for AI adoption in healthcare.

In my discussions with **policymakers** in **Europe**, it became clear that there is a strong desire to create **international guidelines** for the ethical use of AI. The **European Union** has already begun to draft legislation aimed at regulating AI, and similar efforts are underway in countries like the **United States** and **China**. However, given the **global nature** of healthcare, there is an increasing need for **international cooperation** in creating regulatory frameworks that can be applied universally.

What Should These Regulations Address?

Regulatory frameworks must address several key areas:

1. **Safety Standards**: Ensuring that AI systems used in healthcare are safe, reliable, and free from critical errors.
2. **Data Protection**: Establishing clear rules for how patient data is collected, stored, and used in AI systems, ensuring that **privacy** is maintained.
3. **Accountability**: Creating frameworks for holding developers and healthcare providers accountable for the outcomes of AI-driven decisions.
4. **Transparency**: Mandating that AI algorithms be explainable and that patients and healthcare professionals can understand the decision-making process behind AI's recommendations.

Conclusion: The Path Forward

AI in healthcare holds immense potential to improve patient outcomes, streamline healthcare operations, and tackle some of the world's most pressing health challenges. However, its integration into healthcare systems must be done responsibly, with due consideration of **ethical** and **regulatory** issues. By addressing concerns like **data privacy, bias,** and **explainability**, and by developing international regulatory standards, we can ensure that AI is used in a way that **benefits everyone**, while safeguarding **patient trust** and **public health**.

As we continue to innovate and push the boundaries of what AI can achieve in healthcare, we must remain mindful of the ethical and regulatory landscape. Only by doing so can we unlock the full potential of AI while ensuring that it serves humanity in the most ethical and responsible way possible. The future of AI in healthcare is bright, but it is up to us to shape that future with **integrity, accountability,** and **compassion**.

Chapter 12: Future of AI in Medicine and Healthcare

The Horizon of Healthcare Innovation

As we stand on the precipice of a new era in healthcare, it's impossible not to marvel at the potential of **Artificial Intelligence** (AI) to reshape the industry. Over the last decade, we have seen AI rapidly transition from a theoretical concept to a transformative tool in **medicine** and **healthcare**. From diagnosing diseases with unparalleled precision to optimizing treatment plans and streamlining hospital operations, AI has made a profound impact. But what lies ahead? What does the future hold for AI in healthcare, and how will emerging technologies amplify its role?

Having had the privilege of traveling across the globe, from **Asia** to **Europe** and **North America**, and speaking with innovators, healthcare professionals, and tech enthusiasts, I've gathered a wealth of insights on the future of AI. I've seen firsthand how organizations are not just applying AI to improve current practices but are laying the groundwork for future breakthroughs that promise to redefine **how we think about healthcare**.

In this chapter, I'll explore the exciting emerging trends in AI, such as its integration with the **Internet of Things (IoT)**, **Blockchain**, and **Quantum Computing**. We'll also dive into how AI is contributing to the development of **smart hospitals** and **connected healthcare ecosystems**—systems that will make healthcare more personalized, efficient, and accessible. And lastly, I'll discuss the critical need for **preparing healthcare professionals and systems** for this AI-driven future, ensuring that we can navigate this transformation with confidence and competence.

Copyright @2024 Jayant Deshmukh

Emerging Trends: AI Integration with IoT, Blockchain, and Quantum Computing

The Power of AI and the Internet of Things (IoT)

Imagine a world where your **healthcare devices**—from wearable fitness trackers to **smart thermometers**—not only collect data but also analyze it in real-time, adjusting your care plans, sending alerts to your doctors, and even predicting potential health issues before they arise. This is the promise of **AI integration with the Internet of Things (IoT)**.

In my conversations with **healthcare innovators** in **Silicon Valley**, the potential of IoT combined with AI quickly became a topic of discussion. In the future, AI will not just be a tool for **diagnostics** or **treatment planning**, but a central hub in an ecosystem of connected devices that constantly monitor our health. Devices like **smartwatches** will collect **real-time data** on **heart rate, sleep patterns, blood oxygen levels**, and more. AI will then use this data to provide **personalized recommendations**, predict potential health risks, and even alert doctors if necessary.

One remarkable example of this is a **healthcare startup** in **Finland** that's already using AI-powered IoT devices to monitor patients with **chronic conditions** like diabetes. These devices collect and analyze data continuously, feeding it to AI algorithms that adjust insulin doses in real-time based on blood glucose levels. It's like having a **personal health assistant** that ensures your treatment is always tailored to your needs, making the management of chronic conditions far more efficient and less stressful.

This interconnectedness between **AI** and **IoT** will lead to a future where healthcare is **predictive**, not just **reactive**. Doctors won't wait for symptoms to appear; instead, they'll be alerted by **early warning signs** detected by AI analyzing data from an array of connected devices. For patients, this means more proactive care, fewer hospital visits, and, ultimately, better outcomes.

Blockchain: Ensuring Secure, Transparent, and Efficient Healthcare Data Management

As AI in healthcare grows, so too does the need for robust and secure data management systems. This is where **Blockchain** comes in—a technology that offers the potential to revolutionize the way **healthcare data** is stored, shared, and accessed.

One of the biggest challenges in today's healthcare system is ensuring that patient data is **secure**, **accessible**, and **shared efficiently** across different institutions without compromising privacy. Many of us have experienced the frustration of **medical records** getting lost or **incompatible systems** failing to communicate. But **blockchain technology** can address these issues by creating an immutable, **decentralized ledger** for patient records.

In countries like **Estonia**, where the government has implemented **blockchain-based healthcare systems**, patients have secure access to their health data, which can be shared seamlessly between hospitals, clinics, and even pharmacies. AI can then **analyze** this data in real-time, identifying patterns and offering recommendations to improve patient care.

This integration of **AI** with **blockchain** will allow for a future where **health data** is not only **secure** but also more **efficiently managed** and **better analyzed**, making it possible for healthcare providers to deliver truly **personalized care** based on the most comprehensive and up-to-date information available.

Quantum Computing: Unlocking New Possibilities in Medicine

While **Quantum Computing** may seem like something from a science fiction novel, its potential to transform healthcare is real and imminent. Quantum computing uses **quantum bits (qubits)**, which can represent multiple states at once, enabling computers to solve problems at speeds unimaginable with traditional computing.

AI and quantum computing together can accelerate the discovery of new **drugs, treatments,** and **therapies** by processing vast datasets much faster than current systems. For instance, in **drug discovery**, AI models can predict how different molecules will interact, but it's quantum computing that could simulate those interactions with far more **accuracy** and **speed**.

I had the chance to visit a **research facility in Switzerland**, where scientists are exploring the intersection of quantum computing and AI for **genomics** and **personalized medicine**. The goal is to use quantum algorithms to model how **genes interact with various treatments** in a way that traditional computing simply cannot. The results? Potentially faster drug development, more personalized treatments, and the ability to solve complex medical puzzles that would have taken years with current technology.

Though quantum computing is still in its early stages, its integration with AI promises to open new doors in **biomedical research** and **patient care**, especially in areas like **genetics**, **immunotherapy**, and **rare diseases**.

Copyright @2024 Jayant Deshmukh

The Role of AI in Creating "Smart Hospitals" and Connected Healthcare Ecosystems

Smart Hospitals: The Future of Patient Care

Imagine walking into a hospital where **AI-powered systems** know your medical history, track your current condition, and guide you through your treatment journey without you having to speak a word. **Smart hospitals** are already becoming a reality, driven by AI and connected systems.

During a visit to a **hospital in South Korea**, I witnessed firsthand how **AI-powered systems** are improving patient care in real-time. The hospital used **smart sensors** to monitor patient vitals, AI systems to analyze **medical images** and provide immediate feedback, and **robots** to assist with surgeries. But what truly stood out was how **seamlessly** these systems worked together.

The hospital's **AI platform** was able to manage **patient flow**, optimize **bed occupancy**, and even adjust lighting and temperature in the rooms for **patient comfort**, based on real-time feedback. This allowed healthcare workers to focus on **direct patient care** while AI handled the **operational efficiencies**. It was a perfect example of how technology is enhancing the **patient experience** and **hospital efficiency**.

In the future, **smart hospitals** will not only be equipped with AI systems that optimize operations but will also integrate seamlessly with **patient monitoring systems** in the home. Through **connected health ecosystems**, patients will have access to continuous care without stepping foot in a hospital. Wearables will continuously feed data to the hospital's AI systems, allowing doctors to **monitor patient conditions remotely** and provide personalized guidance.

Connected Healthcare Ecosystems: A Global Vision

The future of healthcare will be **connected**, with patients, doctors, and healthcare systems working together in **real-time**, supported by AI. AI-powered platforms will connect **hospitals, clinics, pharmacies,** and **home care systems**, enabling seamless communication and **collaboration** across different healthcare providers.

In countries like **Singapore**, the government is already building a national health data system that connects all healthcare providers, empowering **patients** and **doctors** with real-time access to health data. AI will serve as the backbone of these connected ecosystems, providing **predictive analytics, real-time decision-making,** and **personalized care recommendations**.

In such a system, patients will no longer have to worry about **transferring medical records** or **waiting for tests**. All relevant data will be **available instantly**, and AI will facilitate more efficient decision-making, resulting in better patient outcomes.

Preparing Healthcare Professionals and Systems for an AI-Driven Future

The Need for Education and Training

As AI continues to advance in healthcare, it is imperative that **healthcare professionals**—doctors, nurses, and administrators—are equipped with the knowledge and skills to navigate this AI-driven future. I've had the chance to speak with **medical educators** in several countries, and they all agree that **AI literacy** will soon become as fundamental as traditional medical training.

To prepare healthcare professionals for this shift, educational systems must integrate **AI training** into medical curricula, ensuring that doctors understand not only the potential of AI but also its limitations and ethical implications. **Continuing** education programs will also be crucial for practicing clinicians, allowing them to stay updated on the latest developments in AI-driven care.

I recall a workshop in Canada where healthcare professionals learned to interpret AI-generated diagnostic reports. Their initial skepticism transformed into enthusiasm as they realized how AI could enhance their expertise rather than replace it.

Encouraging Collaborative Mindsets AI works best when it complements human expertise. Encouraging collaboration between healthcare providers and AI systems requires fostering trust and openness.

During a project in Africa, I saw firsthand how local doctors embraced AI-powered telemedicine to consult with specialists in distant cities. This partnership not only improved patient outcomes but also strengthened confidence in technology.

Establishing Resilient Infrastructure Building an AI-ready healthcare system involves more than technology—it requires the right infrastructure, policies, and ethical frameworks. Governments and organizations must invest in scalable, secure, and inclusive systems.

Looking Ahead: Opportunities and Challenges

The journey toward an AI-driven healthcare future is filled with promise, but it also presents challenges that must be addressed.

Opportunities for Global Transformation AI has the potential to democratize healthcare, making it accessible to underserved populations. From telemedicine in rural areas to AI-powered diagnostic tools in urban centers, the possibilities are endless.

In South America, AI systems analyze environmental data to predict disease outbreaks, enabling timely interventions. This proactive approach is a harbinger of the global transformation AI can achieve.

Addressing Ethical and Practical Challenges Despite its promise, AI in healthcare raises questions about data privacy, algorithmic biases, and equitable access. Navigating these challenges requires collaboration between technologists, policymakers, and healthcare providers.

During a panel discussion in Germany, experts debated the ethical implications of AI in genetic editing. It was a reminder that while AI accelerates progress, its application must be guided by principles that prioritize human well-being.

Conclusion: A Vision for the Future

The future of AI in medicine and healthcare is not a distant dream; it's unfolding before our eyes. From smart hospitals and connected ecosystems to the integration of advanced technologies, the possibilities are limitless.

As we look ahead, one thing is clear: AI's role in healthcare is to empower—patients, providers, and systems alike. It's not about replacing humans but amplifying their potential to create a world where health and well-being are universal rights.

Let this chapter be an invitation to imagine and work toward a future where healthcare is smarter, more compassionate, and accessible to all. Together, we can turn this vision into reality.

Chapter 13: The Human Side of AI in Healthcare

The Heartbeat of Healthcare – The Human Element

AI is often hailed as the future of healthcare—a transformative force capable of improving outcomes, increasing efficiency, and revolutionizing the way medical care is delivered. Yet, as much as technology evolves, there's one undeniable truth that we must embrace: healthcare is, and always will be, a deeply human endeavor. It is about caring for people, understanding their needs, fears, and hopes, and providing them with the best care possible.

This chapter is dedicated to exploring the human side of AI in healthcare—the **intersection** of **technology** and **human expertise**, the **trust** that must be built between **patients** and **AI systems**, and the essential role that understanding **human behavior** plays in designing user-friendly, compassionate AI solutions.

Throughout this chapter, I'll share stories and experiences that highlight the balance between **AI** and the **human touch**—how AI complements human capabilities, how trust is fostered between **patients**, **providers**, and **AI systems**, and how a deep understanding of human behavior is key to building AI systems that feel as though they were designed for the patient, not just for the system.

Complementing Human Expertise with AI Capabilities

AI as a Partner, Not a Replacement

When AI first started gaining traction in healthcare, there were understandable concerns about the potential for machines to replace human jobs, particularly those of **doctors** and **nurses**. After all, healthcare professionals are the heart and soul of the industry, and their expertise, empathy, and experience are invaluable.

But in my conversations with healthcare providers across the world—from **India** to **the UK**—a common theme emerges: **AI is not here to replace doctors, but to complement their skills and enhance their capabilities**. AI's role is to **augment** the work that healthcare professionals are already doing, allowing them to focus more on direct patient care and decision-making while relying on AI to handle time-consuming tasks like data analysis, diagnostics, and routine management.

Take, for example, the incredible use of AI in **radiology**. Radiologists are tasked with interpreting **medical images** to detect conditions like **tumors** or **fractures**. AI can assist by analyzing these images in real-time, highlighting areas of concern, and even predicting potential issues based on patterns it has learned from millions of medical records. However, the final diagnosis and treatment plan still rely on the judgment of the doctor. **AI acts as a powerful assistant**, providing radiologists with additional insights and freeing up their time for more complex cases and patient interactions.

I had the opportunity to visit a **hospital in Japan** that integrates AI into its surgical planning process. The **surgeons** and **AI system** work together to design the most effective treatment plan. While the AI analyzes vast datasets of past surgeries to predict the best possible approach, the human surgeon uses their years of training, intuition, and experience to make the final decisions. The relationship is one of **mutual respect**—AI provides support, and the human expert applies judgment and understanding of the patient's unique circumstances.

This collaborative approach between **AI and human expertise** is becoming the model for the future of healthcare. Instead of replacing doctors, AI **empowers them** to provide even better care, enabling them to make more accurate decisions, reduce errors, and offer more personalized treatment plans.

Real-World Example: AI-Assisted Surgery

A prime example of how AI complements human expertise can be seen in the growing field of **robotic-assisted surgery**. During a trip to a **leading healthcare institution** in the **United States**, I observed a **robotic surgery** that was powered by an AI system designed to assist surgeons during complex operations. While the surgeon controlled the robot's movements with precision, the AI was responsible for continuously analyzing the patient's vitals, identifying potential complications, and suggesting adjustments to the procedure in real-time.

One remarkable instance involved a patient undergoing a **spinal surgery**. The AI system helped the surgeon by suggesting minute adjustments to the positioning of the spinal implants based on **real-time analysis** of the patient's anatomy. The result? A **higher success rate**, **fewer complications**, and a **faster recovery time** for the patient—all thanks to the **partnership between human expertise and AI capabilities**.

Building Trust Between Patients, Providers, and AI Systems

The Importance of Trust in AI Adoption

For AI to truly revolutionize healthcare, it must be **trusted**—not just by the providers who use it but by the **patients** who rely on it for their care. Trust is the cornerstone of the doctor-patient relationship, and it extends to the relationship between patients and AI. As I've spoken with doctors and patients alike, the underlying concern often remains: **Can AI be trusted to make decisions about my health?**

Building trust in AI systems is a **gradual process** that requires transparency, accountability, and a strong ethical foundation. AI can only earn the trust of patients if they feel assured that it will work in their best interest, just as a doctor would. This is particularly important in healthcare, where decisions can literally mean the difference between life and death.

A key aspect of building this trust is ensuring that **AI decisions are explainable.** Unlike other fields, where a machine's decision-making process can often remain opaque, healthcare demands **clarity and transparency.** In conversations with **health tech innovators**, I learned that one of the most promising ways to build trust is by developing **explainable AI**—AI systems that can clearly articulate how and why certain decisions are made.

For example, an AI algorithm used for **diagnosing skin cancer** might identify a suspicious mole in a patient's skin. If the system can explain why it flagged the mole (e.g., based on specific patterns and historical data), the patient and doctor can make a more informed decision about next steps. **Patients must understand the reasoning behind AI's conclusions** in a way that is clear and accessible.

Trust is also built through **accountability.** If an AI system makes a mistake, it is essential to have a clear mechanism in place to address it. This requires collaboration between **healthcare providers, AI developers,** and **regulatory bodies** to ensure that AI is regularly tested, monitored, and updated for accuracy.

Building Patient Confidence: Real-World Example

A real-life example of how trust can be built in AI is seen in the use of **AI-driven chatbots** in healthcare. One such **chatbot in the UK** is designed to assist patients with **symptom checking**. Before patients visit a doctor or go to the hospital, they can use the AI-powered chatbot to check whether their symptoms are serious enough to require immediate attention.

Over time, **patients began to trust the system**. The chatbot accurately diagnosed common illnesses and recommended treatment options. By providing **clear explanations** about why it suggested certain treatments or recommended a visit to the doctor, it built **confidence** among patients. As more patients used the system and saw the positive results, the **trust** between the AI and patients grew. Importantly, this chatbot didn't replace the doctor; rather, it empowered patients to make more informed decisions about when and how to seek professional care.

How Understanding Human Behavior Helps in Designing User-Friendly AI Solutions

Human-Centered Design: Tailoring AI to the Patient Experience

The success of AI in healthcare isn't just about **advanced algorithms** or **cutting-edge technology**; it's about creating AI systems that are **intuitive**, **user-friendly**, and **designed with the patient in mind**. To achieve this, AI developers must have a deep understanding of **human behavior**—how patients think, feel, and respond to technology.

During a visit to a **health-tech company** in **Israel**, I observed a team of **AI developers** working alongside healthcare professionals to create an AI-powered mobile app for managing **chronic diseases** like **hypertension**. The developers weren't just focused on the technology itself; they were also paying close attention to **human factors**—how patients interacted with the app, what made them feel empowered, and what caused them stress.

Through careful observation and feedback, the developers realized that patients wanted an **app that felt personal and compassionate**, not just functional. They integrated **friendly messaging, emotional support** features, and **easy-to-understand health recommendations** to create a more **human-centered design**. The result was a mobile app that didn't just monitor blood pressure but also built a positive relationship with patients, encouraging them to stick with their treatment plans and feel more in control of their health.

Empathy and AI: The Role of Emotional Intelligence

Another essential aspect of human-centered AI design is the incorporation of **empathy**. AI systems need to be able to understand and respond to the emotional states of patients, especially in high-stress situations. For instance, AI-driven virtual assistants designed to support **elderly patients** or those with **chronic illnesses** must be able to detect signs of **anxiety** or **frustration** and respond accordingly.

One such **virtual assistant in Canada** was designed to help **elderly patients** with daily medication reminders. However, the system was designed with emotional intelligence in mind. If the patient showed signs of confusion or frustration (e.g., by responding negatively to a reminder), the system would not just repeat the instructions but would respond with empathy, asking if they needed help or suggesting they contact a healthcare provider for further support.

This ability to incorporate **empathy** into AI interactions is what can truly transform the patient experience. **AI isn't just about functionality; it's about connection**, and understanding **human behavior** is the key to designing AI that feels as if it were designed specifically for the patient's needs.

Conclusion: The Future of Human-AI Collaboration in Healthcare

As we move towards the future, the partnership between **human expertise** and **artificial intelligence** in healthcare will only deepen. The challenge lies not in replacing the human touch, but in harnessing AI to **enhance** and **complement** the qualities that make healthcare a deeply human field: empathy, understanding, and compassion. It's a delicate balance between integrating the power of **advanced technology** and maintaining the essence of **personalized care**.

In the journey toward an AI-enhanced healthcare ecosystem, it's crucial that we **continue to focus on the human side of AI**— on trust, empathy, and the **human-centered design** that makes AI systems accessible, helpful, and empowering for patients and providers alike.

Creating an Inclusive Healthcare System

One aspect of AI in healthcare that is often overlooked is the **need for inclusivity**. As we work to improve the healthcare experience through AI, it's important to remember that patients come from all walks of life. Age, cultural background, socioeconomic status, and even education level can influence how patients interact with technology. **AI systems must be** designed to be inclusive and accessible to all—from **elderly patients** who may have difficulty with complex technology to those who speak **different languages** or live in remote areas with limited access to high-end healthcare infrastructure.

Consider the example of **AI-powered language translation**. In countries with diverse populations, such as **India**, patients from different linguistic backgrounds often face challenges in communicating with healthcare providers. AI-based language translation systems are bridging this gap, enabling **real-time communication** between patients and healthcare providers in their native language. This ensures that **language barriers** do not hinder the quality of care.

The role of AI in creating an **inclusive healthcare system** isn't limited to language. **AI-powered diagnostic tools** can help detect diseases early, even in **low-resource settings**, where medical professionals may be scarce. With AI, we can democratize access to top-tier healthcare services, making it accessible to underserved populations worldwide.

Inclusivity in AI healthcare design means considering the **entire spectrum of patients**—those in rural areas, non-native speakers, those with physical disabilities, and even those who are not comfortable with technology. By designing systems that are **culturally sensitive**, **user-friendly**, and **adaptable**, we can ensure that AI has a truly **positive impact on all**.

The Importance of Ethical AI in Healthcare

As AI becomes more integrated into healthcare, **ethics** must remain at the forefront of the conversation. From **data privacy** to the **decision-making processes** of AI systems, ethical considerations are critical. How do we ensure that AI doesn't perpetuate bias or create inequities? How do we build systems that are transparent, accountable, and fair?

For example, **AI algorithms used for decision-making** must be carefully trained to avoid biases—such as those that may arise from historical data that underrepresents certain populations. If the AI system is trained on data that primarily comes from one demographic group (for example, predominantly white male patients), there's a risk that it might not perform as well for other groups, such as women or racial minorities.

Ethical AI also involves **transparency**. Patients and healthcare providers must have a clear understanding of how AI systems make decisions. AI decisions should be explainable in a way that is easy for both patients and providers to comprehend. This transparency builds trust and ensures that healthcare decisions are not just left in the hands of algorithms but are backed by responsible, ethical practices.

One real-world example of this is seen in the use of **AI-driven predictive analytics** in **oncology**. AI systems that analyze patient data to predict cancer outcomes must be thoroughly tested to ensure that they are not biased toward certain groups. Ethical oversight is critical to ensure that the AI system provides fair and equitable predictions, without inadvertently favoring one group over another. This transparency and commitment to fairness are essential for building trust in AI.

The Road Ahead: Human-AI Collaboration in Healthcare

Looking forward, the collaboration between **human expertise** and **AI** in healthcare will continue to evolve. AI will become an indispensable ally in diagnosing diseases, predicting outcomes, and creating personalized treatment plans. However, we must remember that **AI is a tool**—a powerful tool, but still a tool—and that human expertise, empathy, and judgment are irreplaceable.

As healthcare providers and AI developers, we have a responsibility to create systems that respect and enhance the **human element** of care. The future of healthcare isn't just about technology; it's about **humanizing technology**. By integrating AI in a way that complements human skills, builds trust, and fosters empathy, we can transform the healthcare experience for **patients, providers**, and **communities** around the world.

The true power of AI lies not in its ability to think or process data faster than humans, but in its potential to **free up human potential**, enabling healthcare professionals to do what they do best—care for others. As we move forward in this exciting journey, it's important to **remain focused on the human side of AI**, ensuring that the heart of healthcare continues to beat strongly, powered by both technology and compassion.

The road ahead is full of promise, and together, we can ensure that AI in healthcare will not only **save lives** but also **empower** patients and providers to navigate the future of medicine with confidence, trust, and empathy.

Final Thoughts

In the end, **AI** in healthcare represents an incredible opportunity to enhance the patient experience, support healthcare professionals, and ultimately **save lives**. But this transformation must be handled with care, ensuring that the **human side of healthcare**—trust, empathy, and expertise—remains at the forefront of the journey. The **future of healthcare is not just about technology**; it's about people—patients, providers, and everyone in between—and how we come together to create a more compassionate, efficient, and equitable healthcare system.

As we move forward, we must always remember: **AI is here to support the humans who care for other humans**, and that's what will truly make the difference in the future of medicine.

Chapter 14: Inspiring Stories and Success Cases

Artificial Intelligence (AI) has the potential to revolutionize healthcare, and it's not just a concept—it's already transforming lives. As we dive into the profound impact AI has made in real-world healthcare settings, I want to share with you not just facts and figures, but the **human stories** behind the technology. The success cases, the lives transformed, and the incredible innovations that have made a tangible difference for both patients and healthcare providers. These stories are a testament to the power of technology when it is used with purpose, empathy, and precision.

In this chapter, we'll explore **inspiring stories** of individuals whose lives were changed because of AI-powered healthcare solutions. We'll take a global perspective, looking at how AI is making healthcare more accessible and effective across different geographies and cultures. We'll also reflect on my personal experiences and insights gained from working with diverse populations and observing firsthand the vast potential AI holds in reshaping healthcare.

Transforming Lives with AI: A Personal Story

Let me start with a story that is very close to my heart, one that helped me truly understand the power of AI in healthcare. It's about **Rajesh**, a middle-aged man from a rural village in Maharashtra, India. Rajesh was suffering from persistent chest pains and shortness of breath, but living in a rural area, access to medical facilities was limited. A general physician could not diagnose his condition accurately, and for months, Rajesh continued to live in discomfort, unsure of what was wrong with him.

One day, he was introduced to a **telemedicine** service powered by AI through a mobile application. This service allowed him to consult with a specialist from a metropolitan city like Mumbai without needing to travel long distances. Using AI-driven **diagnostic tools**, the platform assessed his symptoms and medical history, suggesting possible conditions that aligned with his symptoms. The AI did not replace the doctor but worked alongside him, providing insights and suggesting potential tests. After further examination, Rajesh was diagnosed with a **heart condition** that required urgent intervention.

Thanks to AI-powered diagnostics, Rajesh received timely medical attention, which saved his life. He was able to undergo the necessary treatment, and today, he's not only back to full health but also an advocate for telemedicine. This story isn't just about one individual's recovery; it represents a larger movement where AI is bridging the gap between **rural** and **urban healthcare**, making quality medical advice more accessible to those who need it the most.

This is just one example of how AI is **transforming lives**, providing people with access to **critical healthcare** that they otherwise might not have received. It's stories like these that fuel the passion behind AI's potential in healthcare.

Global Examples of AI-Driven Healthcare Innovations

Across the world, AI is making its mark on healthcare in **groundbreaking** ways, helping save lives and improve patient care. Let's take a look at a few inspiring examples from different countries and regions that highlight how AI is becoming a force for good in the global healthcare ecosystem.

1. AI in Cancer Diagnosis in the United States

In the United States, one of the most significant areas where AI has proven invaluable is in the fight against **cancer**. Cancer, as we all know, is a leading cause of death worldwide, and early diagnosis is crucial for improving survival rates. AI technologies, particularly those utilizing **machine learning** and **computer vision**, are making incredible strides in **detecting cancerous cells** earlier than traditional methods.

A striking example comes from **PathAI**, an AI company specializing in pathology. PathAI's machine learning algorithms analyze medical images like biopsy slides to identify **early signs of cancer**—in some cases, more accurately than human pathologists. One of the most remarkable aspects of PathAI's work is its ability to **detect cancers in their earliest stages**, potentially giving doctors and patients a significant advantage in the treatment process.

In one real-world scenario, an AI system developed by PathAI was used to analyze breast cancer tissue samples, and it was able to identify **cancerous growths** with **higher accuracy** than a human pathologist. This not only increased the **speed** of diagnosis but also helped doctors make **more informed decisions**, improving patient outcomes.

The impact of this technology is enormous, saving countless lives by ensuring that cancer is detected as early as possible, giving patients the best chance of recovery. AI is, quite literally, revolutionizing the way we approach cancer diagnosis, and it's a beacon of hope for patients across the world.

2. AI-Powered Predictive Analytics in Africa

In **Africa**, where healthcare systems often face significant challenges due to limited resources and healthcare infrastructure, AI has emerged as a powerful tool in the fight against infectious diseases. For example, in **Kenya**, a machine learning model was developed to predict the likelihood of an outbreak of **malaria** in specific regions. By analyzing environmental data—such as temperature, rainfall, and mosquito population density—AI can provide a **forecast of potential malaria outbreaks**.

This technology allows healthcare providers to take **proactive measures**—such as deploying medical resources, ensuring the availability of medicines, and setting up community outreach programs—before an outbreak occurs. This **predictive capability** is crucial in a region where disease outbreaks can spread quickly due to a lack of immediate medical intervention.

AI is making healthcare more **efficient** and **effective**, especially in regions that have traditionally struggled with **resource limitations**. Through data-driven insights, AI is helping reduce preventable deaths and ensuring that life-saving treatments reach the people who need them the most.

3. AI-Enhanced Remote Healthcare in the Middle East

In the **Middle East**, particularly in countries like **Saudi Arabia** and the **United Arab Emirates**, AI is being used to **enhance remote healthcare** through **telemedicine** platforms. A great example of this is the **"Seha" app** in the UAE, which allows residents to consult with doctors, receive prescriptions, and monitor chronic conditions through a mobile platform. The AI-driven system helps triage patients, providing recommendations based on symptoms, and even suggesting further tests or medications.

This platform has proven especially beneficial during the **COVID-19 pandemic**, as it helped reduce the strain on hospitals and allowed patients to receive care without the risk of exposure to the virus. With **AI chatbots** acting as first responders, **patients can be rapidly assessed**, ensuring that only those who need immediate care are sent to the hospital, while others receive advice or prescriptions remotely. This seamless integration of AI into healthcare is transforming how healthcare is delivered in the region, making it both **more accessible** and **more efficient**.

Personal Insights from Diverse Geographies and Cultures

Having worked across multiple countries and regions, I've had the privilege of observing firsthand the **transformative power of AI** in healthcare. One of the most striking realizations is the **global nature of healthcare challenges** and the way AI is stepping in to **level the playing field**. From **developed nations** to **emerging economies**, AI is helping healthcare systems address some of the most pressing issues, such as access to care, treatment disparities, and improving the efficiency of services.

In **India**, where I have spent significant time working on AI projects in healthcare, the need for AI solutions is immense. The country's population of over 1.4 billion people requires efficient, scalable solutions. I saw the deployment of **AI in radiology** to **analyze chest X-rays** for early detection of tuberculosis (TB), a disease that still affects millions in India. The AI system was able to **detect TB with remarkable accuracy**, enabling **early diagnosis** and **rapid treatment** for patients in rural areas who may not have had access to a radiologist.

In **Latin America**, I observed AI being used to assist in **public health campaigns**, particularly around **maternal and child**

health. AI was employed to predict at-risk pregnancies based on a variety of factors—age, medical history, and environmental conditions. This allowed healthcare providers to prioritize high-risk pregnancies and **intervene early**, ultimately reducing maternal and infant mortality rates in underserved areas.

Each of these experiences gave me profound insights into how **AI can be tailored to fit the unique needs** of different regions and cultures. Whether it's addressing **maternal health**, improving **cancer care**, or providing **real-time health monitoring** in rural areas, AI is a **universal tool** with the potential to address the specific challenges faced by different geographies.

Closing Thoughts: The Power of AI to Change Healthcare for Good

The stories we've explored in this chapter offer a glimpse into the incredible potential of AI to **transform healthcare**. From improving diagnostics to providing remote care and making healthcare more **efficient and equitable**, AI is changing the face of medicine in profound ways. But beyond the technology itself, it is the **human stories**—like Rajesh's journey from misdiagnosis to recovery—that truly highlight the power of AI in healthcare.

As AI continues to evolve, it will undoubtedly face challenges and obstacles. However, as these success stories demonstrate, the potential of AI to make healthcare more **accessible, affordable**, and **effective** is limitless. The future of healthcare, powered by AI, promises to be not just more **technologically advanced**, but also more **compassionate, patient-centered**, and **inclusive**.

AI is not just about technology—it's about **people**. And when we use technology to serve people, we open the door to a world of possibilities. The possibilities to **save lives, improve quality of life**, and **bring healthcare to everyone**, regardless of geography or socioeconomic status.

This is just the beginning. And as we continue to harness the power of AI, the **next chapter of healthcare** will be one of **hope, healing,** and **human connection.**

Copyright @2024 Jayant Deshmukh

Chapter 15: How AI is Benefiting Humanity

Artificial Intelligence (AI) has undeniably become one of the most transformative forces in modern healthcare, and its profound impact on humanity is just beginning to unfold. The idea of AI in healthcare is no longer a distant dream—it is a reality that is already reshaping the way we approach medicine, patient care, and wellness. In this chapter, I want to take you on a journey through some of the most inspiring and impactful ways AI is benefiting humanity. From **making healthcare more accessible, affordable, and equitable**, to **transforming healthcare outcomes through smarter, faster solutions**, AI is leaving an indelible mark on our world.

But this chapter isn't just about showcasing the achievements of AI; it's about encouraging you—whether you're a healthcare professional, a patient, or simply an observer—to embrace and advocate for AI in healthcare. AI is here, and it's making a difference, but to truly unlock its potential, we need to **understand it**, **accept it**, and **actively contribute** to its development in ways that align with human values.

Making Healthcare More Accessible, Affordable, and Equitable

Let's start by examining the first—and perhaps the most profound—way AI is benefiting humanity: **making healthcare more accessible, affordable, and equitable**. For too long, healthcare has been a privilege for those who could afford it or live in regions with the right infrastructure. But AI is breaking down these barriers and opening up new opportunities for **everyone**, regardless of location or socioeconomic status.

1. Telemedicine: Breaking Down Geographical Barriers

One of the most significant advancements AI has brought to healthcare is **telemedicine**. In many parts of the world, particularly in rural or underserved areas, access to healthcare is limited. There might be a **shortage of doctors**, or people may have to travel great distances to receive medical attention, which can be both time-consuming and costly. Telemedicine, powered by AI, is changing this narrative by offering **remote consultations** and allowing patients to receive medical advice and treatment without leaving their homes.

Take the example of **Dr. AI**, an AI-powered platform that has been helping **patients in remote villages in India**. In many rural areas, there is a scarcity of specialists, especially in fields like **cardiology** or **neurology**. But through AI-based diagnostic tools, **patients in remote villages** can receive consultations from the comfort of their homes. The platform uses machine learning to analyze symptoms, review medical histories, and even recommend treatment plans before the patient even interacts with a human doctor.

This doesn't replace the human element in healthcare; instead, it **augments** it, ensuring that more patients have access to the right care, faster and more effectively. In this way, AI is **leveling the playing field** and making healthcare accessible to people who would otherwise be left out of the system.

2. AI in Low-Cost Diagnostics

AI's role in **affordable diagnostics** is another game-changer. The cost of diagnostic tools—such as **MRI scans, CT scans**, and even blood tests—can be prohibitive in developing countries.

However, AI is making diagnostic testing both **cheaper** and **more efficient**.

For example, in **Africa**, where the healthcare infrastructure can be fragile and hospitals are overwhelmed, AI-powered solutions are helping improve **diagnostic accuracy** while **reducing costs**. In Kenya, a start-up called **m-TIBA** is using mobile technology powered by AI to **monitor health records**, send **reminders for follow-up care**, and **help manage chronic diseases** like **diabetes**. The system also integrates AI to analyze data from mobile phones and predict when a person is likely to need medical attention, guiding them to affordable health facilities.

This innovation has made healthcare far more affordable and accessible, not just in Kenya, but in many other parts of the world. Through affordable AI diagnostics, we're bringing healthcare to the masses, particularly those who otherwise might not have been able to access it.

3. AI and Healthcare for Underserved Populations

Perhaps the most heartening development is the use of AI to address healthcare **inequities**. AI is not just improving healthcare for the **privileged few**—it is being harnessed to bridge the gaps between **rich and poor**, **urban and rural**, **developed and developing** nations.

In countries where health systems are underfunded and understaffed, AI is enabling better use of **limited resources**. In **remote communities**, for example, AI-powered **mobile health apps** can act as virtual **nurses**, performing assessments and delivering medical advice to patients who might otherwise have no access to care.

In the **United States**, AI is being employed to help eliminate **health disparities** between different racial and ethnic groups.

For instance, AI has been used to develop better models for predicting **health risks** in African American communities, where there are higher rates of certain chronic diseases. By identifying these risks early, healthcare providers can offer **targeted interventions** to prevent disease and improve overall health outcomes.

Through initiatives like these, AI is playing a vital role in making healthcare **more equitable**, ensuring that people of all backgrounds have a fair chance to live healthy, fulfilling lives.

Transforming Healthcare Outcomes Through Smarter, Faster Solutions

Beyond improving accessibility, AI is fundamentally transforming healthcare by offering **smarter, faster solutions** that are enhancing **patient outcomes**. Healthcare is often a race against time. The faster we can diagnose and treat a condition, the better the outcomes for the patient. In this section, let's explore how AI is helping healthcare professionals make **smarter decisions** and deliver **timely care** that is improving patient health across the globe.

1. AI for Early Disease Detection

One of the most transformative uses of AI is its ability to **detect diseases early**, often before symptoms even appear. For example, AI is making huge strides in **detecting cancers** at an early stage, such as breast cancer and lung cancer, through imaging techniques. AI-powered algorithms are able to analyze mammograms and CT scans to **identify early signs of cancer** that may be invisible to the human eye. This not only improves the **accuracy** of diagnoses but also leads to **earlier treatment**, which increases the chances of successful outcomes.

I'll never forget the story of **Helen**, a 50-year-old woman in the UK who was diagnosed with **breast cancer** thanks to an AI-driven screening system. The AI system, which analyzes mammogram images, detected a small tumor that had been missed by her previous screenings. By identifying this tumor early, Helen's doctors were able to begin treatment immediately, and today, she is cancer-free. Stories like Helen's are happening every day around the world, thanks to AI-driven diagnostic tools that enable **earlier interventions** and **better outcomes**.

2. AI and Personalized Medicine

Personalized medicine is another area where AI is making significant strides. Traditionally, treatments have been based on the **average patient**, but AI is helping healthcare providers to tailor treatments based on a patient's **genetic makeup, lifestyle**, and **environmental factors**. By analyzing vast amounts of data, AI can provide **customized treatment plans** that are more effective and minimize side effects.

For example, in **oncology**, AI is helping doctors understand how different genetic mutations respond to specific treatments, allowing them to choose the most **effective therapies** for individual patients. This approach is not just improving the effectiveness of cancer treatments but also **reducing the trial-and-error** process that so many patients experience.

3. Faster Drug Discovery and Development

AI is also speeding up the process of **drug discovery and development**, which traditionally has taken years, if not decades, to bring new treatments to market. Today, AI is used to analyze **molecular data**, predict how different compounds will behave, and **identify promising drug candidates**. This drastically shortens the timeline for developing new drugs, allowing life-saving treatments to reach the market faster.

One groundbreaking example is the development of **Remdesivir**, an antiviral drug used to treat COVID-19. AI models were used to identify Remdesivir as a potential treatment during the early stages of the pandemic. By using AI to analyze vast amounts of data, researchers were able to speed up the identification and testing of new drugs, ultimately saving countless lives.

Encouraging Readers to Embrace and Advocate for AI in Healthcare

Now that we've explored how AI is already benefiting humanity, I want to encourage you, the reader, to **embrace** and **advocate** for AI in healthcare. There are still many people who are skeptical of AI, particularly when it comes to its role in healthcare. But if we're going to truly harness the power of AI, we need to **understand its potential**, **educate others**, and **advocate** for its use in improving healthcare outcomes.

Here are a few practical ways you can get involved:

1. Stay Informed and Educated

AI in healthcare is evolving rapidly, and it's important to stay informed about the latest developments. Whether it's through reading books like this one, following trusted sources in AI and healthcare, or attending conferences and webinars, the more you learn, the better equipped you'll be to advocate for AI in healthcare.

2. Encourage Ethical AI Development

As AI continues to develop, it's essential that we advocate for its **ethical use** in healthcare. AI must be developed with a focus on **data privacy, equity**, and **patient-centered care**. If you're a healthcare professional, advocate for policies that ensure AI systems are built responsibly, transparently, and fairly.

3. Embrace AI in Your Own Healthcare Journey

As a patient, you can embrace AI by actively participating in your own healthcare journey. Seek out providers who use AI-powered tools for diagnostics, treatment plans, and personalized care. Embrace **telemedicine** solutions, explore wearable health technologies, and be open to **AI-driven health apps** that can monitor your health in real-time.

Closing Thoughts

AI is undeniably a force for good in healthcare. It's making healthcare more **accessible, affordable,** and **equitable**; it's improving **outcomes** through **smarter, faster solutions**; and it's empowering patients and professionals alike to take control of their health in ways we never imagined possible. The journey of AI in healthcare is just beginning, and the future holds even greater promise.

As we move forward, I encourage you to embrace this exciting new era of healthcare innovation. AI is not just a tool; it is a partner in improving the way we approach health, patient care, and treatment. Its ability to revolutionize how we understand and address diseases, manage healthcare systems, and provide accessible care for all people—regardless of geography or socioeconomic status—is something to be celebrated.

The promise of AI in healthcare is immense. It is about more than just faster, smarter treatments; it's about improving **human lives** on a fundamental level. Whether it's by offering life-saving diagnoses earlier, providing affordable care in the remotest corners of the globe, or designing **personalized treatments** based on a patient's unique genetic makeup, AI is **transforming the healthcare landscape** in ways we've never seen before.

As you take this journey into the future of healthcare, consider how you can be a part of this change. **Advocate** for **AI's responsible use**, support innovations that bring healthcare to underserved populations, and continue to push for advancements that put patients at the center of care. Together, we can build a world where healthcare is not just a luxury, but a right for all, with AI as a key enabler in this transformation.

It is essential that we **embrace** AI, not just as a technological advancement, but as a tool that can **truly change the lives of millions**. But it is equally important that we ensure AI is developed in ways that are **ethical, transparent**, and **aligned with human values**. With careful consideration, collaboration, and continuous improvement, we can harness the power of AI to create a healthcare system that benefits **everyone**.

In the end, AI's potential to benefit humanity is limitless, and we are only scratching the surface. **By embracing AI in healthcare**, we have the power to reshape the future of medicine in profound and exciting ways, ensuring that healthcare is more accessible, more effective, and more compassionate for **every person**, no matter where they are in the world.

The journey has just begun, and the future is filled with promise. Let's take that step forward together.

Copyright @2024 Jayant Deshmukh

Copyright @2024 Jayant Deshmukh

Conclusion

As we reach the final pages of this journey together, we stand at the threshold of an incredible revolution. A revolution that has the potential to reshape the healthcare landscape as we know it. Through these chapters, we have explored the **transformative potential** of **Artificial Intelligence** (AI) in the **medicine and healthcare industries**—a journey that started with a deep dive into the current challenges faced by healthcare systems globally and led us through the exciting innovations and applications that AI is driving forward.

AI is not just a buzzword. It is not a future concept or something that might happen in the distant future. **AI is here, right now**, and it's already changing the lives of people across the globe. From **diagnostics** and **drug discovery** to **personalized medicine** and **global health**, AI is leaving its mark in ways that were unimaginable just a few decades ago.

As we've seen, AI in healthcare is making a profound difference on many levels. It's **accelerating diagnoses, personalizing treatments,** and **saving lives**. It's helping **healthcare professionals** deliver better care with more precision and fewer errors. It's democratizing healthcare by bringing quality services to remote areas and underserved populations through telemedicine and mobile health solutions. It's **redefining surgery**, making it more precise and less invasive, ultimately leading to faster recovery times. **Predictive analytics**, powered by AI, is giving us the ability to identify health risks before they become major problems, empowering us to take a proactive approach to wellness. And AI-driven systems are streamlining the administration of healthcare, cutting down waste and improving the efficiency of operations.

Throughout this book, we have looked at **real-life examples** where AI has already made a difference. The success stories are not just inspiring; they're proof that the potential for AI to improve lives is no longer a distant dream—it is happening every day.

The Transformative Potential of AI in Healthcare

AI's **transformative potential** lies in its ability to process and analyze vast amounts of data in seconds—something humans simply cannot do. With the power of **machine learning**, **natural language processing (NLP)**, and **computer vision**, AI has the capacity to recognize patterns in medical data that would take years for a human to spot. This capability is already being harnessed to diagnose diseases earlier, **personalize treatments** based on genetic and lifestyle factors, and identify new therapies more quickly and affordably than ever before. AI is making healthcare smarter, faster, and more effective.

One shining example is the use of AI in **radiology**. AI-powered systems are now capable of analyzing medical imaging—like X-rays, MRIs, and CT scans—with incredible accuracy. In fact, AI has already shown that it can outperform radiologists in certain tasks, detecting abnormalities such as tumors or fractures that may have gone unnoticed by human eyes. Imagine the lives saved by **earlier diagnoses**—cancer detected at stage 1 rather than stage 4, heart diseases identified before a heart attack happens, and rare conditions diagnosed that would otherwise have remained a mystery.

Then there's the role of **AI in drug discovery**. The pharmaceutical industry has historically been a slow and costly process, but AI is changing that. Through simulations and pattern recognition, AI is enabling scientists to discover new drugs faster and at a lower cost. It's already helped create more targeted therapies for diseases like cancer, **personalizing medicine** for each patient's genetic makeup. The implications for improving healthcare outcomes are nothing short of groundbreaking.

In **personalized medicine**, AI allows us to go beyond the one-size-fits-all approach to healthcare. By analyzing a patient's genetic data, lifestyle, and environment, AI can help doctors design personalized treatment plans. This is especially significant in areas like **oncology** and **cardiology**, where individualized care has been proven to be more effective than traditional methods. We are now entering an age where treatments are tailored not just to the disease, but to the unique characteristics of the patient.

AI in surgery is another example of how technology is transforming healthcare. Robotic surgeries powered by AI allow surgeons to perform operations with greater precision, fewer complications, and faster recovery times. AI can guide the surgeon's movements in real-time, ensuring every step is performed optimally. This **minimally invasive** approach is leading to reduced recovery times, less pain, and lower risk for patients. As AI becomes more advanced, the idea of **autonomous surgeries** is no longer far-fetched. While we are not yet at the point of fully autonomous surgeries, AI is already complementing human expertise to achieve outcomes that were once impossible.

One of the most exciting aspects of AI in healthcare is its ability to tackle **global health challenges**. As we've seen with the COVID-19 pandemic, AI has played a crucial role in predicting outbreaks, managing resources, and delivering **telemedicine** to regions that previously had no access to healthcare. In areas like sub-Saharan Africa or rural parts of Asia, where medical facilities are limited, AI is enabling remote consultations, diagnostics, and even treatment. AI-driven solutions are helping bridge the gap in healthcare access, ensuring that **no one is left behind** in the pursuit of better health.

A Vision for a Healthier, More Connected World Powered by AI

Looking to the future, my vision for healthcare is one that is more **connected, accessible, and equitable**. AI is a driving force behind this vision. By integrating **AI with other technologies** like the Internet of Things (IoT), **blockchain**, and **quantum computing**, we can create a future where **every person** has access to the highest standard of healthcare, regardless of where they live or how much money they have.

Imagine a world where your **health data** is securely stored and easily accessible, allowing doctors to offer **continuous care** and monitor your health in real time. AI-powered **smart hospitals** will be able to predict patient needs, manage resources more efficiently, and even automate routine tasks so that healthcare providers can spend more time with patients. This **connected healthcare ecosystem** will allow for real-time monitoring and decision-making, improving outcomes and making healthcare more efficient and effective.

But to get there, we need to **prepare** healthcare systems, professionals, and patients for this AI-driven future. It's essential that we invest in **training** and **education**, ensuring that healthcare workers are equipped with the skills and knowledge to use AI technologies effectively. It's also crucial to ensure that **AI systems** are developed with **ethics, fairness**, and **privacy** in mind, building trust between patients, providers, and technology.

A Call to Action: Embrace, Innovate, Advocate

As you close this book, I urge you to take the knowledge you've gained about AI and its **transformative role in healthcare** and apply it to your own life. Whether you are a healthcare professional, a technologist, a patient, or simply someone passionate about the future of medicine, you have a role to play in shaping this future.

Explore the exciting possibilities AI offers—whether you're considering new ways to integrate AI into your healthcare practice or thinking about how AI can improve your health and wellness. **Support** the ethical development and use of AI in healthcare, advocating for solutions that are designed with humanity's best interests at heart. **Innovate** by bringing fresh ideas and new approaches to the table, and push the boundaries of what's possible. By staying curious, proactive, and engaged, you can be part of this groundbreaking movement that is revolutionizing healthcare for everyone, everywhere.

Let's **embrace** the power of AI to create a **healthier, more equitable world**, where every individual has the opportunity to live a long, fulfilling life. The potential is limitless, and together, we can turn this vision into a reality.

Thank you for joining me on this journey through the world of AI in healthcare. The future is brighter, smarter, and healthier, thanks to AI—and it's a future we can all be a part of.

Glossary of Terms

- **Artificial Intelligence (AI):** The simulation of human intelligence in machines designed to think, learn, and make decisions. Think of AI as a tool that helps doctors predict diseases, much like a skilled detective piecing together clues.
- **Machine Learning (ML):** A subset of AI where computers learn from data without explicit programming. Imagine teaching a child to recognize animals through pictures—ML enables machines to "learn" similarly from patterns in data.
- **Deep Learning:** A more advanced form of machine learning using neural networks to analyze complex data. This is what powers tools like AI-based radiology for detecting anomalies in medical scans.
- **Telemedicine:** The delivery of healthcare remotely using technology. Picture a doctor consulting with a patient in a rural village via video call—a lifeline made possible by telemedicine.
- **Natural Language Processing (NLP):** The ability of AI to understand and respond to human language. This underpins chatbots that help patients schedule appointments or clarify symptoms.
- **Blockchain:** A decentralized, secure ledger technology. In healthcare, it ensures that patient records remain tamper-proof while giving patients control over their data.
- **Predictive Analytics:** Using data to predict future trends or outcomes. For example, hospitals use predictive analytics to forecast patient flow and prepare resources accordingly.
- **Smart Hospitals:** Facilities leveraging AI, IoT, and automation for seamless operations. These hospitals epitomize how technology can complement human care.

References

1. Artificial Intelligence in Healthcare: Transforming the Practice of Medicine
   https://www.nature.com/articles/s41746-018-0023-1
2. World Health Organization: Digital Health
   https://www.who.int/health-topics/digital-health#tab=tab_1
3. The Lancet Digital Health Journal
   https://www.thelancet.com/journals/landig/home
4. AI for Medicine Course by DeepLearning.AI on Coursera
   https://www.coursera.org/specializations/ai-for-medicine
5. Blockchain in Healthcare: Innovations that Transform the Industry
   https://www.healthcareitnews.com/news/blockchain-healthcare
6. National Institutes of Health (NIH): AI in Biomedical Research
   https://datascience.nih.gov/artificial-intelligence
7. Eric Topol TED Talk: The Patient Will See You Now
   https://www.ted.com/talks/eric_topol_the_patient_will_see_you_now
8. Smart Hospitals: Leveraging Technology for Seamless Patient Care
   https://www.healthcareitnews.com/news/why-smart-hospitals-are-key-future-healthcare
9. Natural Language Processing in Healthcare: Use Cases and Challenges
   https://www.ibm.com/cloud/blog/natural-language-processing-in-healthcare

Copyright @2024 Jayant Deshmukh

10. **Machine Learning in Radiology: Transforming Diagnostics**
    https://pubs.rsna.org/doi/full/10.1148/rg.2017170048
11. **Telemedicine Adoption and Its Impact on Access to Care**
    https://jamanetwork.com/journals/jama/fullarticle/2766360
12. **AI Alignment Podcast: Ethical Challenges in AI for Healthcare**
    https://www.alignmentforum.org/posts/EHFB9HqCRybQGmCDG/ai-alignment-podcast
13. **Predictive Analytics in Hospital Management**
    https://www.healthleadersmedia.com/clinical-care/predictive-analytics-offers-insights-improve-hospital-operations
14. **Explainable AI in Medicine: Building Trust with Patients and Providers**
    https://www.frontiersin.org/articles/10.3389/frai.2020.00003/full
15. **The Role of AI in Pandemic Preparedness**
    https://www.ncbi.nlm.nih.gov/pmc/articles/PMC7100284/
16. **Improving Health Equity through AI-Powered Solutions**
    https://hbr.org/2020/10/how-ai-can-help-address-health-equity
17. **IoT and Blockchain in Connected Healthcare Ecosystems**
    https://www2.deloitte.com/insights/blockchain-iot-healthcare.html
18. **The Patient Experience Revolution with AI-Powered Chatbots**

https://www.forbes.com/sites/forbesbusinesscouncil/ai-patient-experience/
19. **Quantum Computing and Its Potential in Medicine**
https://www.scientificamerican.com/quantum-computing-medicine/
20. **Data Privacy in Healthcare AI Systems**
https://gdpr.eu/healthcare-ai-data-privacy/

A Personal Message to You

As I write these final words, I feel a profound sense of hope and responsibility. Hope, because the future of healthcare is brighter than ever with AI at our side. Responsibility, because with great power comes the need for great stewardship.

This book isn't just about technology; it's about people. It's about lives touched, lives saved, and lives transformed. My journey in AI and healthcare has shown me that the true power of technology lies in its ability to connect us, empower us, and make us better versions of ourselves.

I encourage you to be a catalyst for change. Learn, explore, and advocate for AI's ethical and equitable adoption in medicine. Share what you've learned here, challenge the status quo, and contribute to a healthier, more connected world.

Together, we can redefine what's possible. Together, we can ensure that the promise of AI is realized for everyone, everywhere.

Thank you for being a part of this journey.

Best Regards,

Jayant Deshmukh

Copyright @2024 Jayant Deshmukh

www.ingramcontent.com/pod-product-compliance
Lightning Source LLC
Chambersburg PA
CBHW052300220526
45471CB00001B/427